MW01115478

HERBAL ANTIBIOTICS

What BIG Pharma Doesn't Want You to Know

How to Pick and Use the 45 Most Powerful Herbal Antibiotics for Overcoming Any Ailment

By Mary Jones

Copyright© 2016 by Mary Jones – All rights reserved.

Copyright: No part of this publication may be reproduced without written permission from the author, except by a reviewer who may quote brief passages or reproduce illustrations in a review with appropriate credits; nor may any part of this book be reproduced, stored in a retrieval system, or transmitted in any form or by any means – electronic, mechanical, photocopying, recording, or other – without prior written permission of the copyright holder.

The trademarks are used without any consent, and the publication of the trademark is without permission or backing by the trademark owner. All trademarks and brands within this book are for clarifying purposes only and are owned by the owners themselves.

Disclaimer: The information in this book is not to be used as professional medical advice and is not meant to treat or diagnose medical problems. The information presented should be used in combination with guidance from a competent professional person.

The information in this book is true and complete to the best of our knowledge. All recommendations are made without guarantee on the part of the author. It is the sole responsibility of the reader to educate and train in the use of all or any specialized equipment that may be used or referenced in this book that could cause harm or injury to the user or applicant. The author disclaims any liability in connection with the use of this information. References are provided for informational purposes only and do not constitute endorsement of any websites or other sources. Readers should be aware that the websites listed in this book may change.

First Printing, 2016 – Printed in the United States of America

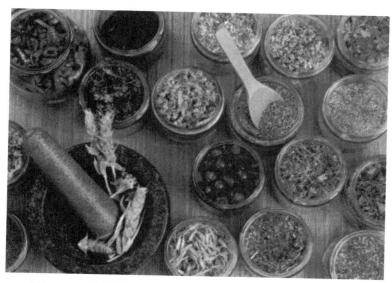

"Healthy people eating healthy food should never need to take an antibiotic"
– Joel Fuhrman, American author, physician, speaker

TABLE OF CONTENTS

INTRODUCTION

Herbal antibiotics – among other medicines – have been used by healers for centuries to ward off a wide range of ailments. These natural remedies have steadily become more popular in recent years, and *are very close to becoming a mainstream treatment.* This is because bacteria have become resistant to man-made products, and it's only by returning to the more natural ingredients, that we can rebuild immunity to them.

This guide will look at **how to ward off illness and infection using these herbal remedies**, and the abundance of benefits that you will experience from switching. Once you have read all of the data contained in the chapters below, you will never look back!

An antibiotic has been defined by medicinenet.com as: *"A drug used to treat infections caused by bacteria and other microorganisms. Originally an antibiotic was a substance produced by one microorganism that selectively inhibits the growth of another. Synthetic antibiotics, usually chemically related to natural antibiotics, have since been produced that accomplish comparable tasks."*

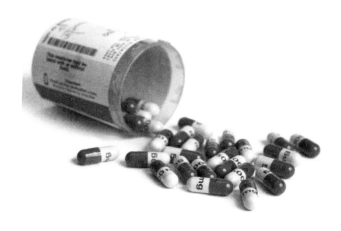

Antibiotics were originally compounds made from all-natural ingredients — before they became the liquid or pill we know them as today. There are many common ingredients in these herbal medications, ones that you may recognize.

The fifteen most common are:

- Acacia
- Aloe
- Cryptolepis
- Echinacea
- Eucalyptus
- Garlic
- Ginger
- Goldenseal
- Grapefruit Seed Extract
- Honey
- Juniper
- Licorice
- Sage
- Usnea
- Wormwood

To find out more about how these work within the medications, and how they can be beneficial to you, please read on. This is the most extensive guide on this topic that you'll be able to find. All the information is offered as a guideline; you must consult your doctor before using these remedies.

CHAPTER 1
CONTROVERSIAL FACTS ABOUT BACTERIA

Bacteria may only consist of a single cell, but they are amazingly complex. Most of us know bacteria as '*germs*,' invading our bodies and making us ill, but actually they co-exist with us a lot of the time helping to maintain our atmosphere. In fact, there is over one million types of bacteria that live in your body, in your intestines, on your skin, and even on your genitalia. These are known as 'good bacteria,' and do not cause disease – they are actually good for our health.

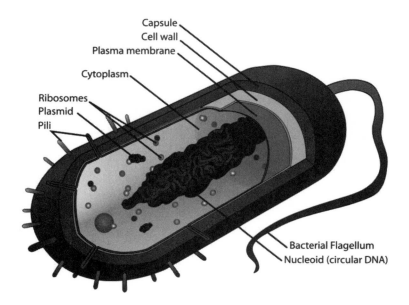

That being said, **bacteria *can* lead to illness**. A report conducted by the *Center for Disease Control* (CDC) in 2011 found that 1 in 6 Americans – 48 million people – get sick from foodborne diseases caused by bacteria, 128,000 are hospitalized, and 3,000 people die.

Top five pathogens contributing to domestically acquired foodborne illnesses

Pathogen	Estimated number of illnesses	90% credible interval	%
Norovirus	5,461,731	3,227,078–8,309,480	58
Salmonella, nontyphoidal	1,027,561	644,786–1,679,667	11
Clostridium perfringens	965,958	192,316–2,483,309	10
Campylobacter spp.	845,024	337,031–1,611,083	9
Staphylococcus aureus	241,148	72,341–529,417	3
Subtotal			91

Top five pathogens contributing to domestically acquired foodborne illnesses resulting in death

Pathogen	Estimated number of deaths	90% credible interval	%
Salmonella, nontyphoidal	378	0–1,011	28
Toxoplasma gondii	327	200–482	24
Listeria monocytogenes	255	0–733	19
Norovirus	149	84–237	11
Campylobacter spp.	76	0–332	6
Subtotal			88

The most common diseases that are caused by bacteria are:

- *Helicobacter pylori* can cause ulcers and gastritis.
- *Neisseria gonorrhoeae* can cause gonorrhea (sexually transmitted disease).
- *Neisseria meningitides* can cause meningitis.
- *Salmonella* and *Escherichia coli* (*E.coli*) can cause food poisoning.
- *Staphylococcus aureus* can lead to various infections in the body, such as abscesses, boils, cellulitis, food poisoning, toxic shock syndrome, and wound infections.

- *Streptococcal bacteria* can lead to various infections in the body, such as ear infections, pneumonia, strep throat, and meningitis.

The four main types of bacteria that can cause illness:

- *Bacilli* – shaped like a rod with a length of around 0.03 mm. Causes illnesses such as typhoid and cystitis.
- *Cocci* – shaped like a sphere with a diameter of approximately 0.001 mm. Cocci bacteria can arrange themselves in pairs, long lines, or tight clusters, causing diseases such as staphylococci and gonococci.
- *Spirochaetes* – shaped like a tiny spiral, these bacteria cause illnesses like syphilis.
- *Vibrio* – shaped like a comma, they cause diseases like cholera.

Bacterial diseases such as these are highly contagious and often result in severe life-threatening issues, including toxic shock syndrome, blood poisoning, and kidney failure. Even though the symptoms associated with these diseases can vary, *a very classic sign of a bacterial infection is fever.* You will likely experience chills, headaches, ear pain, a rash, lesions, fatigue, a stiff neck, vomiting and nausea, irritability, diarrhea, abdominal pain, bloody urine, a sore throat, coughing, chest pain, abscesses, weight loss, muscle spasms, joint pain, and body aches.

The first step to curing these diseases is via prevention. There are vaccinations available for some bacterial diseases, such as meningitis, pneumonia, tetanus, and rabies. You can also be sure to wash your hands and cover your mouth when you cough to prevent the spread, but if you manage to get one anyway, you are likely to be prescribed with antibiotics.

There are alternative treatments to help with bacterial diseases – **herbal antibiotics that can help you fight off these infections**. The following remedies are recommended:

- *Probiotics* – they increase the body's good bacteria and reduce the function of the bad ones. They are great for treating bacterial vaginosis, intestinal and stomach infections, etc.
- *Aloe Vera* – aloe vera, usually in gel form, has been extracted from the plant and can be used as a treatment for internal infections, such as urinary and vaginal infections or bacterial skin infections, etc.
- *Turmeric* – turmeric powder combined with milk is great for respiratory infections due to the high antioxidant content of curcumin.
- *Apple Cider Vinegar* – great for many bacterial infections in the body because it maintains your body's pH balance.

- ***Tea Tree Oil*** – very effective for a host of skin and vaginal bacterial infections.
- ***Garlic*** – cloves of garlic can be a treatment for respiratory, urinary, and digestive infections, plus bacterial infections of the skin.
- ***Ginger*** – ginger enhances blood circulation, which makes it a good treatment for stomach and respiratory infections.
- ***Honey*** – organic honey soothes dry coughs and irritated throats when consumed with warm water or ginger tea.
- ***Baking Soda*** – great treatment for skin infections; make a paste by adding to warm water. Baking soda also works by restoring the body's pH balance.
- ***Lemon*** – removes bacteria by reducing the mucus build-up from inside the respiratory tract.
- ***Cranberry Juice*** – an effective treatment for urinary tract and vaginal infections that can be taken several times daily to overpower the bad bacteria.

Suggestions for dealing with bacterial infections:

General guidelines: Stop consuming dairy, sugar, alcohol, refined foods, meat, and caffeine. Regularly consume hot, warm, and room temperature beverages, for example, herbal tea, and eat lightly. Water or juice fasting for a couple days and taking enemas can help you fight an infection by flushing your system. Add zinc, beta carotene, and Vitamin C supplements to your diet, which can help strengthen your immune system. Echinacea and goldenseal also boost your immune system. Detox your system with steam baths, saunas, and massages, such as a foot massage with garlic oil. Get plenty of rest, pay attention to what your body is telling you, and don't push yourself if you're sick. It could take your body even longer to recover.

Throat: Natural remedies can be effective treatments for throat infections, such as strep throat, which is diagnosed by taking a throat culture, but it's also very important to confirm with a blood test that there is no lingering strep. When undetected, it can generate joint, heart, or kidney problems. Try herbal throat lozenges or gargles – salt water, bitter orange oil, goldenseal, myrrh, or calendula – to alleviate throat infection symptoms. Homeopathy, applying mercurius, belladonna, Phytolacca, Lycopodium, or Lachesis, can be an effective treatment for throat infections, as well. An unusual, and lesser known, remedy Spigelia can provide relief from strep throat symptoms within forty-eight hours.

Skin: Skin infections can be bacterial and fungal. Apply a mixture of St. John's wort tincture and calendula to a bacterial skin infection. Apply homeopathy, diluted vinegar, turmeric powder, and tea tree oil topically to fungal skin infections. Other typically used herbs are plantain, goldenseal, and comfrey. Cysts and boils can be effectively treated with homeopathic remedies – *Hepar sulphuris* and silica – Epsom salt soaks, a ginger poultice, and hot packs.

Bladder: Treat a bladder infection immediately! There will be more pain, and an increased risk of kidney infection, if you wait too long. Then you could end up requiring traditional antibiotics. Drink plenty of water and cranberry juice, or take cranberry capsules; take herbs (including Berberis, goldenseal, buchu, uva ursi, and Chimaphilia); and apply homeopathy (including the remedies sarsaparilla, staphisagria, Apis, and Cantharis).

Sinuses: Consume hot ginger tea and avoid dairy. Try applying an effective Ayurvedic mixture called *Sitopaladi* to break up mucus congestion. There are effective homeopathic remedies, as well, that include onion (*Allium cepa*), Kali bichromicum, salt (*Natrum muriaticum*), Pulsatilla, and mercurius. Taking a steam bath, using a sauna, or employing the Neti Pot and warm salt water to irrigate your sinuses can also be effective treatments.

CHAPTER 2
ANTIBIOTIC RESISTANCE

Antibiotic resistance is defined as bacteria becoming resistant to drugs or being able to survive exposure to antibiotic medications. These become known as *'Multi Drug Resistant'* (MDR) or more commonly *'Superbugs.'* The most well-known of these superbugs is **MRSA** *(Methicillin Resistant Staphylococcus Aureus)*.

The superbugs' resistance to drugs may be based on acquiring resistance genes among other bacteria or mutation. Although, it can also be attributed to the widespread use of antibiotics. Our bodies have become so used to using them, that they no longer have the desired impact on our immune systems.

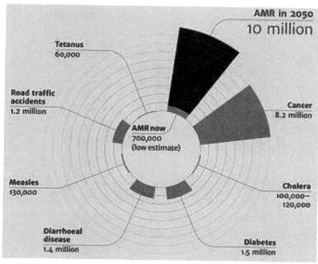

AMR = Antimicrobial Resistance

On April 30, 2014, a report by the *World Health Organization* made the following **guidelines to counteract antibiotic resistance**:

- *Only* use antibiotics after they are prescribed by your doctor.
- Complete the full course of antibiotics, even if you feel better.
- Never use leftover antibiotics or share them with others.

Although antibiotic misuse is a major factor in drug-resistant bacteria, there are other **things you can do daily to help the prevention of this**:

- Be sure to wash your hands before and after using the toilet, blowing your nose, changing diapers, and food handling.
- Always cover your nose and mouth while sneezing and coughing, and never spit.
- Always use, and then properly dispose of, tissues to wipe and blow your nose.
- Keep yourself at home when you feel ill, and keep your children at home if they are ill.
- If you still feel unwell after your course of antibiotics, return to the doctor for help.

The number of diseases earning the **'superbug'** title increases over time, but at this current time, **the following list is relevant**:

- *Staphylococcus Aureus (MRSA)* – in 1947, penicillin resistance was found in MRSA, which is found on the human skin and mucous membranes. Now, this disease is quite common and is responsible for many hospital fatalities.
- *Streptococcus* and *Enterococcus* – these need a combination of antibiotics to get rid of them. Streptococcus is responsible for arthritis, meningitis, sinusitis, pneumonia, peritonitis, bacteremia, and otitis media.
- *Pseudomonas Aeruginosa* – this is a highly prevalent opportunist pathogen. It has a low antibiotic susceptibility.
- *Clostridium Difficile* – a pathogen originating in hospitals causing diarrheal disease. Some studies suggest that *Clostridium difficile* is down to the overuse of antibiotics in livestock.
- *Salmonella* and *E.coli* – these are often the result of drinking contaminated water. They have become more dangerous, with more fatalities, due to the widespread use of antibiotics.

- *Acinetobacter Baumannii* – on November 5, 2004, the CDC reported an increasing number of sufferers in medical facilities or among the soldiers who had fought in Iraq or Kuwait.

- *Klebsiella Pneumoniae* – this is an emerging bacterium that is extremely drug-resistant and Gram-negative. The rapidly increasing incidence of this bacillus in clinical settings worldwide is troubling because it causes infections known to have high mortality and morbidity rates.

- *Mycobacterium Tuberculosis* – multidrug resistant tuberculosis (TB) is responsible for 150,000 deaths every year. TB had no cure until Selman Waksman discovered streptomycin in 1943; it was a very common and easily spread disease until then. It didn't take long for the bacteria to develop a resistance, which occurs due to spontaneous genome mutations. Recently, the drugs Rifampin and Isoniazid have been applied as treatments.

- *Neisseria Gonorrhoeae* – this pathogen is transmitted via sex and may cause vaginal and penile discharge, painful urination, and pelvic pain, along with other systemic infection symptoms. Records of the bacteria suggest that it was identified as early as 1879. Treatment with penicillin was effective in the 1940s, but a drug-resistant strain developed in the 1970s.

These superbugs often have to be treated with a combination of powerful antibiotics. Experts and scientists are working constantly to discover the weakness in these viruses, to give them a suitable chance at fighting them.

Here is an important quote from one of the scientists who has dedicated their work to this: *"Discovery of a fungus capable of rendering these multidrug-resistant organisms incapable of further infection is huge,"* says microbiologist and infectious disease specialist, Irena Kenneley, from Cleveland's Case Western Reserve University and the Frances Payne Bolton School of Nursing. *"The availability of more treatment options will ultimately save many more lives."*

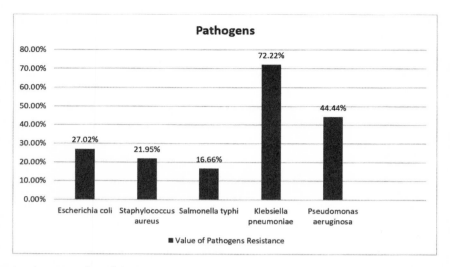

As the use of antibiotics in farming (which promotes growth and prevents infection in the animals) has contributed to the mutation of drug-resistant infections, one way to give yourself a better chance is to only consume meat that has been raised on organic farms.

There are other, more **natural ways, that you can use to assist your immune system in the fight against these bacteria**, and they include:

- *Tea Tree Oil* – which has a proven ability to fight off and kill staph bacteria. It's used as a topical application, going directly on infected skin.

- *Apple Cider Vinegar and Baking Soda* – the mix of these two ingredients can make a paste, which works in a similar way to tea tree oil.

- *Garlic* – the complex makeup of garlic is great for fighting infections and enhancing your immune system.

- *Coriander Oil* – a study in 2011 by Portuguese scientists found that coriander oil is effective against twelve lethal bacteria.

- *Pascalite* – can bring total recovery to wounds by drawing infection out when applied topically. This cousin to bentonite clay can only be found in the mountains of Wyoming.

- *Turmeric* – a healing product that, for centuries, has been used to fight viral and bacterial infections. It has proven anti-inflammatory and antibacterial properties.

- *Manuka Honey* – treatment for MRSA and other superbugs when combined with turmeric.

- *Oil of Oregano* – it has a proven ability to fight bacteria and staph infections.

- *Olive Leaf Extract* – combats antibiotic-resistant infections and supports the immune system at the same time.

- *Echinacea* – has the ability to fight most severe bacteria, even though it is mostly used today against colds and flu. Traditionally has been used to treat syphilitic lesions, open wounds, blood poisoning, diphtheria, and cellulitis.

- *Colloidal Silver* – well-known killer of viruses, bacteria, and fungal infections. For over a century, compounded with anecdotal evidence and clinical cases, colloidal silver has been applied for its antibacterial and germicidal properties.

- *Pau D'arco* – this South American herb has an active ingredient, lapachol, that can relieve a variety of infections, such as those caused by fungus, viruses, and bacteria.

So, as you can see, although there are no known cures for these superbugs at this current time, there are things we can do to protect ourselves, and help us fight off these bacteria, with both traditional and herbal medication.

CHAPTER 3

EYE-OPENING ALTERNATIVE MEDICINE STATISTICS

NCCAM – the National Center for Complementary and Alternative Medicine – is the federal government agency that conducts scientific research for alternative medicine. On their website at <u>nccam.nih.gov</u>, the following claims are made:

Our Mission:

The mission of NCCAM is to define, through rigorous scientific investigation, the usefulness and safety of complementary and alternative medicine interventions and their roles in improving health and health car.

Our Vision:

Scientific evidence informs decision making by the public, by health care professionals, and by health policymakers regarding use and integration of complementary and alternative medicine.

A lot of their research shows what and how complementary and alternative medicine is used. The diagrams below show the findings of this data (CAM = *Complementary and Alternative Medicine*):

COMPLEMENTARY & ALTERNATIVE MEDICINE
— Popularity & Uses

Complementary & Alternative Medicine (CAM):

Treatment that is used in addition to (complimentary) or instead of (alternative) traditional treatments. Typically complementary and alternative treatments are more natural, and less invasive than traditional treatments. These treatments can range from natural supplements to chiropractic adjustments to Qi gong and yoga.

HOW POPULAR ARE
Complementary & Alternative Medicine?

38%
of American adults use CAM

12%
of American children use CAM

WHAT IS
CAM
COMMONLY
Used To Treat?

NECK PAIN
5.9%

BACK PAIN
17.1%

ARTHRITIS
3.5%

JOINT PAIN
5.2%

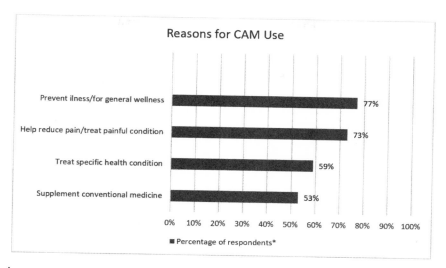

*Base: Respondents who used CAM in past 12 months or ever (n=539). Sampling error = 4.2 percentage points. Respondents could choose more than one answer.

Source: AARP/NCCAM Survey of U.S. Adults 50+, 2010

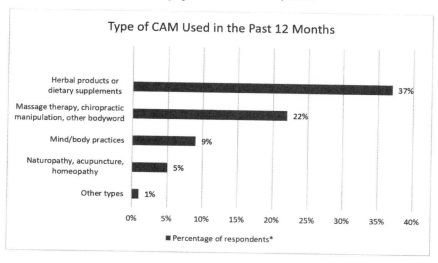

*Base: All respondents (n=1013). Sampling error = 3.1 percentage points. Respondents could choose more than one answer.

Source: AARP/NCCAM Survey of U.S. Adults 50+, 2010

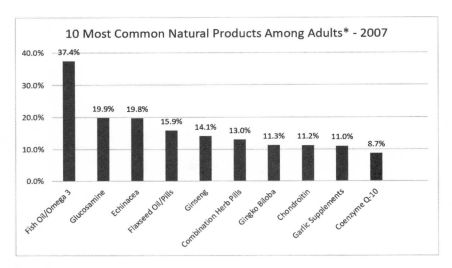

*Percentages among adults who used natural products in the last 30 days.

Source: Barnes PM, Bloom B, Nahin R. CDC National Health Statistics Report #12. Complementary and Alternative Medicine Use Among Adults and Children: United States, 2007.

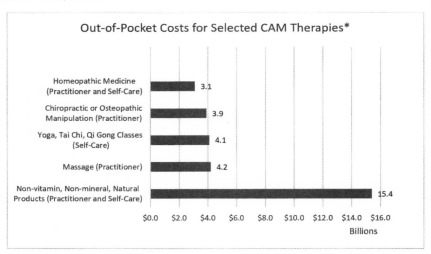

Totals for non-vitamin, non-mineral, natural products and homeopathy include both — CAM practitioner costs and costs of purchasing CAM products. Totals for massage and chiropractic manipulation are only for CAM practitioner costs. Totals for yoga, tai chi and qi gong classes are only the costs of purchasing CAM products.

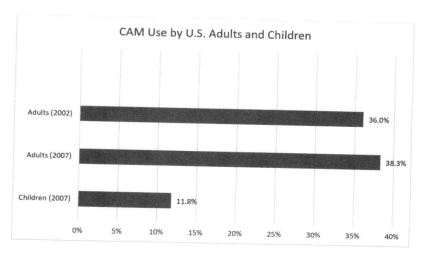

Source: Barnes PM, Bloom B, Nahin R. CDC National Health Statistics Report #12. Complementary and Alternative Medicine Use Among Adults and Children: United States, 2007.

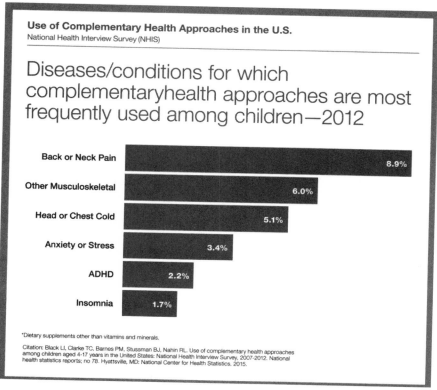

A study into '*Public Perceptions of Herbal Medicines*,' which Ipsos MORI conducted for the MHRA (*Medicines and Healthcare products Regulatory Agency*) in 2008, conducted a research program.

The results of this were fascinating, and demonstrate just how we are becoming more content to use herbal therapies to avoid all of the side effects experienced from traditional medication. When asked about **words associated with herbal medication**, the most common were:

- Safe
- Natural
- Non-addictive
- Pure

Which demonstrates that, generally, people have a positive view of their usage and do not seem to pose any threats to users. Some of the **quotes from the research groups**, when asked what herbal medication was, were as follows:

"To me, it means something that's been grown or produced without any chemicals in it."

"And non-addictive. They're supposed to be non-addictive."

"A few years ago when I was breastfeeding I had to take mixed pollen for my hay fever, and I got the idea that the herbal medicines build up your resistance more, and maybe that's why it takes longer to work."

These broad statements demonstrate how little we actually know about herbal medication and the benefits we can receive from them. By not researching the information available and trusting traditional medication solely, we are not giving our bodies the opportunity to discover what more natural remedies can do for us.

"The condition I have is a hormonal one and it affected my skin, and twice I've been treated with the NHS treatment, which is the strongest treatment in the world that you can take, and the side effects were horrific. It wasn't worth it, and I still to this day feel physically ill because of what I took. I think it's a really dangerous NHS drug and it's been known to push people to commit suicide, and I thought I can't, I'll never, ever take that again, it's too risky. And I went to the Chinese medicine and it's worked for me and with no side effects."

"I was in China a few years ago and I watched a man, in fact I filmed him burn his own hands on a red hot chain and then he applied herbal cream to his hands. ...And when he wiped his hands clean there were no marks on his skin. ...I believe that there are a lot of medicines, herbal medicines that would work. But I think most of it is we don't do it because we're ignorant of it."

As these two contrasting statements show, the biggest barrier people face when looking at herbal medication is information. We have doctors and pharmacists that are more than happy to discuss traditional medication, but it's more difficult to obtain facts about how natural medications work – which is why this guide has been created.

The facts about herbal antibiotics

The antibiotics that your doctor prescribes are synthetic. One of the scary problems facing mainstream medicine is the increase in antibiotic-resistant bacteria. What is most concerning is that there are some bacteria that have developed a resistance to almost all antibiotics. Bacteria can genetically adjust for an antibiotic and transfer the resistance to other bacteria very rapidly.

So how are herbal antibiotics any better? It's because herbal antibiotics are more complex.

Penicillin is one compound. But garlic, as an example, contains 33 sulfur compounds, 17 amino acids, and more! So while it's easier for bacteria to mutate and become resistant to a single compound, it's much more difficult for them to mutate for a complex herbal antibiotic.

From this, it's easy to see the benefits of herbal medication and why more people are turning to it on an annual basis. The NCCAM data below shows the age range of people using complementary and alternative medicine, and due to all the information shown so far, this is due to continue to grow dramatically.

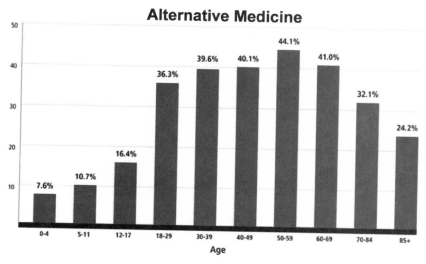

CHAPTER 4
USAGE OF ANTIBIOTICS –
ALL YOU NEED TO KNOW

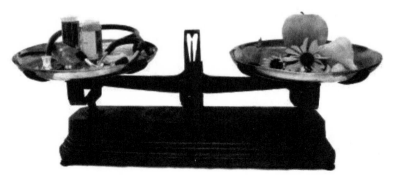

The choice to use herbal antibiotics is a very personal one. As demonstrated in the last chapter, having all of the information is pivotal to making the lifestyle change to using herbal medications – and this includes antibiotics. You have to be sure that they are right for you. Of course, in emergency situations, such as acute illness or trauma, you cannot fault the work of traditional antibiotics. What herbal medication works better for is **prevention**, **chronic disease**, and the **after effects** left behind by these antibiotics.

A study presented at <u>umm.edu/health/medical/altmed/treatment/herbal-medicine</u> shows that nearly one-third of Americans use herbal remedies. Although there are ***things you will want to consider***, ensuring that they are the right fit for you and your health:

- *Other medication that you are taking* – you will need to consult with your doctor to check that they don't interact badly.

- *Side effects* – although herbal medication has much less possibility of side effects than conventional antibiotics, you still need to learn what the possibilities are in case they affect you.

- *Regulation* – herbal medication isn't regulated in the way that conventional treatments are. There are a lot of resources and information available for you to make your own decisions, but there are a few groups that haven't been properly tested on – women who are pregnant or breastfeeding, children, or the elderly.

Infections can be described in two parts '*heat*' and '*damp*.' It suggests that antibiotics are brilliant for treating the 'heat' part of the infection – fever, sore throat, inflammation – whereas, they often leave the 'damp' symptoms – phlegm, nausea, foggy-headedness – alone. This is why many herbalists will often recommend herbal treatments alongside the conventional medicine.

Antibiotics are primarily used for bacterial infections, such as:

- Moderately severe acne, or not especially serious conditions, but they will not likely clear up without antibiotics.

- Impetigo skin infection or chlamydia (sexually transmitted infection), or not especially serious conditions that could spread to other people if left untreated.

- Kidney infection, or conditions where antibiotics could help decrease recovery time based on evidence.

- Pneumonia or cellulitis, or conditions with the risk of generating more serious complications.

The creation of antibiotics began in 1877, when Louis Pasteur discovered that saprophytic bacteria repressed the growth of the anthrax disease. Then, in 1928, the most important contribution to the world of antibiotics occurred when Alexander Fleming made the discovery that led to penicillin. Since the 1970s, synthetic modifications of any naturally occurring antibiotics have been provided as new antibiotics.

The process of creating antibiotics is **fermentation**. If you're interested in this process, the steps are listed below:

1. Isolate the desired organism that will produce the antibiotic and increase its numbers many times. Do this by creating a starter culture in a lab, which is taken from a sample of the organism that had been isolated and cold-stored. Transfer that organism sample to an agar-

containing plate to grow the initial culture. Then, the initial culture and food and nutrients are put into shake flasks for growth. From this process, a suspension is created, which will be transferred to seed tanks.

2. Seed tanks are made of steel and designed to sustain an ideal growing environment. They have been filled with the things a specific microorganism requires to survive and thrive. For example, carbohydrate-based foods – such as glucose sugars or lactose – and warm water and growth factors including minor nutrients, amino acids, and vitamins. Also, the seed tanks need to include additional necessary sources of carbon: nitrogen sources, acetic acid, hydrocarbons, or alcohols. These tanks have also been equipped with mixers to keep moving the growth medium and a pump that delivers filtered, sterilized air. The material in the seed tanks will be transferred to primary fermentation tanks after about 24-28 hours.

3. Fermentation tanks can hold up to 30,000 gallons. Essentially, it is a larger version of the seed tanks. They are providing an environment that sustains growth by being filled with the same growth content found in the seed tanks. The microorganisms will multiply and grow here. It is during this process where the large quantities of the antibiotic are excreted. The temperature of the tanks are maintained between 73-81° F (23-27.2° C). A stream of sterilized air is constantly pumped into the tanks, and the contents are constantly agitated. Due to this, agents to prevent foaming will be periodically added. Additionally, acids and bases are added as necessary to maintain pH control, which is vital for optimal growth.

4. The isolation process begins after three to five days, when the maximum amount of antibiotic has been produced. The fermentation broth can be processed with any of a variety of purification methods, specific to the antibiotic being created. For instance, for water-soluble antibiotic compounds, an ion-exchange method might be employed. Otherwise, for an oil-soluble antibiotic, for example penicillin, a solvent-extraction method might be employed. In either case, when this step is complete, the manufacturer ends up with a purified antibiotic in powdered form. This can be refined further to generate different products.

5. Antibiotics are offered in various forms. They are applied as powders in topical ointments, pill or gel-capsule form, and as solutions for syringes or IV (intravenous) bags. A variety of refining steps could be taken post-initial isolation; this will depend on the antibiotic's final form. For powdered versions, the ointment and antibiotic are mixed directly. When used in capsule form, powdered antibiotic is added to the bottom of the capsule and the top half is mechanically connected. If the solution is being added to intravenous bags, crystalline antibiotic

will get dissolved into a solution and added to the bag that will be hermetically sealed.

6. Now the final product can be transported to its final packaging station. The products will be stacked, then loaded into boxes. After being put on distribution trucks, they will be delivered to pharmacies, hospitals, and distributors. This whole process from fermentation to processing could take as long as five to eight days.

These **antibiotics work by making effective use of the differences between the composition of the host's cell and the bacteria's cell**. They either kill the bacteria entirely or keep the cells from multiplying, which leave their number the same allowing the body to fight them off with its natural defenses.

These antibiotics can be delivered in one of three ways:

- *Orally* – drinkable liquids, pills, capsules, or tablets used as a treatment for most types of mild to moderate body infections.

- *Topically* – drops, creams, sprays, or lotions often used as a treatment for skin infections.

- *Injections* – drip infusion or an injection applied directly to the muscle or in the blood, which are typically reserved for severe infections.

Synthetic antibiotics can be divided into six different categories:

- *Penicillins* – widely used as a treatment for various infections, including urinary tract, skin, and chest infections.

- *Cephalosporins* – used as a treatment for a range of infections. Also effective as a treatment for severe infections, including meningitis and septicemia.

- *Aminoglycosides* – used as a treatment for serious illnesses, including septicemia, because they have potentially serious side effects, such as kidney damage and hearing loss. They can be applied as drops, for eye or ear infections, and injection because of how quickly the digestive system can break them down.

- *Tetracyclines* – used as a treatment for a variety of infections. Commonly, it has been used to combat rosacea (spots and flushing of the skin) and severe acne.

- *Macrolides* – used in the treatment of chest and lung infections. Also provided as an alternative to penicillin, for people with an allergy, or in the treatment of penicillin-resistant bacteria strains.

- *Fluoroquinolones* – used as a treatment for a wide range of infections, because they are considered broad-spectrum antibiotics.

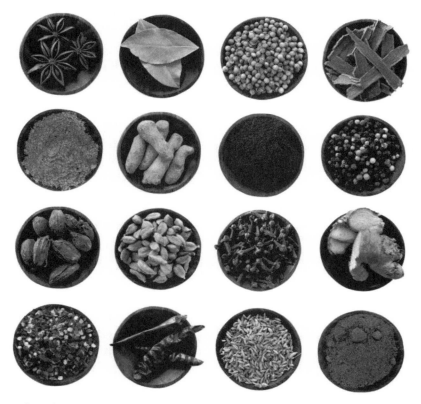

But what about the more natural, **herbal antibiotics**? How do you decide **which ones are right for you**? Well, there are plenty of places you can get information from, and your doctor or pharmacist is one of these sources. Of course, they may try and encourage you to stick to traditional medication, but if you stick by your guns, they will be extremely useful in telling you what you can and can't take due to your current medication list. Of course, to decide whether or not the herbal medication is for you – once you know that they are safe for you to take – the best thing you can do is try them. Once you've tried the recommended dosage, you'll know how effective they are for your body.

Several factors will determine how effective an herb will be. Natural herbs contain a variety of ingredients, and how they work together may have a beneficial effect. In several instances, scientists can't pinpoint the specific ingredient in a specific herb that is working to treat an illness or condition. Even the growth environment (soil quality, harvesting and processing, bugs, or climate) will have an effect on how or why it works.

Natural antibiotics work in two ways: they *eliminate dangerous* *germs*, and they ***boost the body's natural defenses***. Several foods, spices, and herbs have the needed natural, antibiotic qualities to help combat certain ailments.

Some examples with information on how they work are listed below:

Oregano Oil

Oregano essential oil is considered potent enough to combat a variety of microorganisms, especially when tested against similar oils. Oregano oil contains carvacrol and thymol, which are two potent antifungal, antibacterial constituents. They can help prevent secondary bacterial infections. Oregano oil might also be effective in the treatment of urinary tract infections, gastrointestinal disorders, respiratory tract disorders, and menstrual cramps. Research has determined it can also fight staph infections (*Staphylococcus aureus*), and it works when applied topically to control skin conditions, such as dandruff or acne.

Honey

Even though honey has effective, inherent anti-inflammatory properties, not every type of honey works the same way. For example, the New Zealand-native Manuka honey contains the chemical compound methylglyoxal (MG). It is believed that MG is what gives Manuka its active antibacterial properties. Because Manuka can treat wounds, it is sterilized and packaged as a medical-grade honey.

Garlic

Garlic has been applied as an antibacterial for a long time. Typical usage includes treatment for high blood pressure, common cold and the flu, and warts and fungal skin infections. There is potential, based on garlic's properties, for treating diabetes, some cancers, and even heart disease. In fact, when facing penicillin shortages during World War II, several Russian medics applied garlic in its place.

Tea Tree Oil

Tea tree oil is used as an antiseptic against skin conditions such as athlete's foot and acne, fungal infections, as well as herpes and vaginal infections, and ear and mouth infections. Extracted oil from the *alternifolia* species of the *Melaleuca* tree has proven the most effective to fight certain types of bacteria, and it is not as irritating to your skin.

Elderberry

Recent research has emphasized an immune-boosting property from elderberry juice and other water-based extracts. It is also active in destroying free radicals, which works to protect your cells from damage inflicted by disease and infections. These black or blue berries have antioxidant benefits that can fight tonsillitis, some cancers, and coughs, colds, and flu and that assist in lowering bad cholesterol.

Berberine

Berberine is a naturally occurring chemical within several herbs, such as goldenseal and Oregon grape, offering broad-spectrum properties that are similar to antibiotics. Recent research found that both goldenseal extract and berberine can help fight influenza. Traditional Chinese and Ayurvedic medicines have made use of this chemical for a long time. Berberine is widely used for its antimicrobial properties, fighting against bacterial (for example, bacterial diarrhea), viral, and fungal infections (for example, eye infections), along with worms and protozoans.

Andrographis

Based on various human clinical trials, andrographis is one of the best immune-boosting herbs. It is commonly used to fight upper respiratory tract infections by alleviating the severity of its symptoms – sore throat, fever, nasal discharge, expectoration, disturbed sleep, headache, fatigue/malaise, and earache.

Herbal remedies are also brilliant for dealing with the side effects left behind by antibiotics:

- Chronic sinus congestion
- Fatigue, heaviness, or fogginess
- Recurrent sinus or bladder infection
- Urinary urgency or pressure
- Chronic yeast infection
- Loose stools, bloating, or loss of appetite
- Nausea or sickness
- Abdominal pain or diarrhea

Here are some **complementary treatments** to look after your body while you're using antibiotics:

- *Probiotics* – rebuild the body's good bacteria.
- *Herbal Tea* – to help combat nausea.
- *Milk Thistle* – for the antioxidant effects on your liver.

You should also be:

- Eating onion and garlic to support your liver and to keep your yeast in check.
- Taking Omega 3, Vitamins C and E, and Oregon grape root.
- Ensuring that you consume a well-balanced diet.

Of course, it is important to keep the pros and cons of antibiotics and more natural remedies in mind. These need to be considered when making your decision on what to take.

Pros of Antibiotics

These are some of the advantages of using antibiotics:

- They *can treat a wide variety of infections*, including sinusitis, strep throat, and tonsillitis.

- They can be *taken orally or by injection*, making most antibiotics easy to administer.

- They have *minor side effects*, making many antibiotics the perfect option for the times you are extremely sick.

- They are *cost-effective*, making most older antibiotics, and generic alternatives, more affordable – especially, when you can't afford health insurance.

Cons of Antibiotics

You should also be aware of the disadvantages of antibiotics:

- They may cause *allergic reactions*, making it more difficult to find an effective treatment for your illness.

- There may be *drug-resistant bacteria*, making it difficult to treat bacteria remaining in your system when you don't take the full dose. This means antibiotics could not be as beneficial for you in the future.

- There may be *negative side effects*, making effective antibiotics harder to find. Some negative side effects might be nausea and digestion issues, diarrhea, sensitivity to light, or general discomfort.

On top of this, a Finnish study demonstrates that the effects of antibiotics on intestinal bacteria were still visible after a year. This means that the after effects of antibiotic use are damaging for a long time. The continual overuse of antibiotics will lead to more strains of drug-resistant bacteria developing and more unnecessary deaths will occur, which is why we should use herbal antibiotic treatments wherever possible.

Pros of Natural Remedies

The advantages of using herbal remedies rather than pharmaceuticals:

- *Lower risk for side effects.* Herbal remedies tend to be better tolerated by a patient. There are fewer unintended effects with an herbal remedy than with pharmaceutical products. It is more likely that herbs will be safer to apply over a long period of time. For example, Vioxx is a well-known pharmaceutical in the treatment of arthritis, where herbs used for treatment have a lower risk for major side effects. Due to an increased risk of patients suffering cardiovascular issues, Vioxx was recalled. On the other hand, alternative treatments for arthritis generated few side effects. Those treatments included specific dietary modifications, such as slowing down consumption of white sugar, increasing consumption of simple herbs, and avoiding vegetables from the nightshade family.

- *Better results for chronic conditions.* Herbal remedies have an established history of being more effective with long-standing health issues that are resistant to traditional or pharmaceutical medicines.

- *Manageable prices.* Herbs typically cost much less than their pharmaceutical counterparts. The costs of prescription or pharmaceutical remedies inevitably include the costs for researching, testing, and then marketing those drugs.

- *Easier accessibility.* Herbs are always available everywhere; sometimes being accessible at your nearest grocery store – without ever needing a prescription. Depending on the herbs you need for remedies, there is the possibility of growing them right in your home, popular examples are chamomile and peppermint. There are remote regions in the world where the only medicine accessible for the majority of people is herbal remedies.

Cons of Natural Remedies

Herbs may not be appropriate in every situation, and they have other disadvantages to remember:

- *Not appropriate in treating certain conditions:* Herbal remedies and alternative treatments are not as effective in treating accidents or serious and sudden illnesses as modern medicinal treatments. Traumas, such as a broken leg, appendicitis, or a heart attack, could not be treated as effectively by an herbalist as a traditional medical practitioner using drugs, surgery, or modern diagnostic tests.

- *No specific dosage guidelines:* There is a very real risk for doing harm to yourself by self-dosing with herbs. The risk for overdose is so great, and probable, because herbs typically do not come with the inserts or instructions that accompany prescription or pharmaceutical remedies.

- *Wild herbs come with a poison risk:* When people try to identify and then harvest wild herbs, they take a, admittedly foolhardy, risk. If one uses the wrong part of the plant or misidentifies it entirely, there is a very real risk of unintentionally poisoning themselves.

- *Potential interaction with current medications:* It is very important to discuss any new herbal remedies with your current doctor, because herbs can and will interact with your current medications. For example, herbs applied to alleviate anxiety, including St. John's wort and Valerian, do interact with prescription antidepressants.

- *No government regulation or oversight:* Consumers run a very real risk of buying low-quality herbs because these products are not given government regulation or oversight. Herb quality can vary among brands, batches, or manufacturers. This inconsistency can make prescribing the proper dose of each herb that much more difficult.

From these lists, it's clear to see why herbal antibiotics have been used for centuries – for a long time before synthetic antibiotics were created. They work alongside our bodies to fight off bacteria and infection, which is why we are left with far fewer side effects. Even if you need to take prescription antibiotics, herbal remedies are great for keeping your body healthy and combating any side effects that may occur.

CHAPTER 5

HOW TO FIGHT
INFECTIONS NATURALLY

There are many ways that your body can fight infections and strengthen your immune system naturally – it is designed to do so. Sometimes it just needs a little help when bacteria has mutated. Aside from herbal medication, there are **factors that you can include in your everyday lifestyle** as preventative methods:

- Stop smoking.

- Maintain a balanced diet.

- Work out regularly.

- Stay at a healthy weight.

- Monitor your blood pressure.

- Only drink alcohol in moderation.

- Make sure you get enough sleep.

- Take the steps, for example, washing hands and thoroughly cooking meat, to prevent infection.

- Get regular medical check-ups and screenings.

There are many different herbs that contain antibiotic qualities – many of which are discussed in detail in the next chapter – and there are some **key essential oils** that you should be aware of.

Essential oil	Major constituent (content)	Distributor
Cinnamon bark oil	cinnamaldehyde (63.1%)	La Florina (Germany)
Lemongrass oil	neral (33.2%), geranial (37.8%)	Sanoflore (France)
Perilla oil	limonene (18.9%), perillaldehyde (60.8%)	Kohken Koryo (Japan)
Thyme (wild) oil	carvacrol (80.0%)	Neal's Yard Far East (Japan)
Thyme (red) oil	limonene (25.8%), γ-terpinene (19.4%), thymol (25.5%)	La Florina (Germany)
Thyme (geraniol) oil	geraniol (32.7%), geranyl acetate (55.6%)	Sanoflore (France)
Peppermint oil	p-menthone (19.5%), menthol (63.5%)	Sanoflore (France)
Tea tree oil	γ-terpinene (17.7%), terpinen-4-ol (42.5%)	Thursday Plantation (Australia)
Coriander oil	linalool (73.2%)	Sanoflore (France)
Lavender (spike) oil	1,8-cineole (23.7%), linalool (46.3%), camphor (17.1%)	Sanoflore (France)
Lavender (true) oil	linalool (30.1%), linalyl acetate (36.6%)	Sanoflore (France)
Rosemary oil	α-pinene (24.1%), 1,8-cineole (23.5%), camphor (19.7%)	Sanoflore (France)
Eucalptus (radiata) oil	1,8-cineole (74.3%), α-terpineol (10.3%)	Sanoflore (France)
Citron oil	limonene (83.1%)	Kohken Koryo (Japan)

Content of each major constituent was determined from a peak area relative to the total peak area in GC analysis. Major constituents of >15% content are listed here, with the exception of eucalyptus oil. Multiple constituents are arranged in the order of retention time in GC.

Another study (at anandaapothecary.com/articles/antibacterial-essential-oils.html) lists the most well-known essential oils as thyme, tea tree, lavender, oregano, geranium, and lemon. This second study looks further into what is popular, rather than scientific fact, but both are equally relevant.

Many antibiotics can be found in *food, herbs, and spices*. The following is the list of most useful:

Food:

- Honey
- Cabbage
- Fermented Foods
- Horseradish
- Lemon
- Pineapple
- Curd
- Turmeric
- Ginger
- Carrot
- Onions and Garlic

Herbs and Spices:

- Thyme
- Mints
- Basil
- Cinnamon Sage

- Chervil
- Rosemary
- Lemon Balm
- Oregano
- Cumin Tarragon
- Cloves
- Bay Leaf
- Chili Peppers
- Marjoram
- Caraway Seed
- Coriander
- Dill
- Nutmeg
- Cardamom
- Pepper

CHAPTER 6
TOP 45 WONDROUS HERBS

1. Onions and Garlic

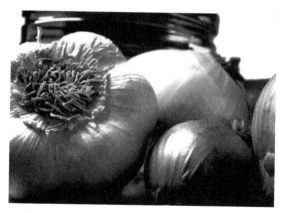

Garlic and onion have been used to help combat the residual effects of the flu and colds. As the antifungal properties of garlic work to prevent yeast infections and fight off viral conditions, the high phytonutrient content in onions clear away free radicals that may lead to cancer. Research was conducted where mice were tested with garlic against an antibiotic-resistant strain of *Staphylococci*. Results revealed that garlic significantly reduced inflammation and protected the mice against the pathogen.

TIP: Did you know about onion's magnetic power? It attracts all germs and bacteria. If a person falls ill, keep an onion bulb under his feet. You can also place some onion pieces near that person. They will draw all the toxins from the body.

Availability: Can be purchased from most food-based shops. (e.g. iHerb.com, Amazon.com, naturesbest.co.uk)

Antibiotic Properties: The sulphur compounds in onions and garlic are a key ingredient in antibiotics. They destroy bad bacteria and kill off infections. *Primarily used for lowering blood pressure, also for diabetes.*

Collection & Preparation: Available as powder, tablets, capsules or can be consumed in food (preferably raw).

Dosage: 2-5 g of powder per day or take it raw.

Possible Side Effects: The smell can often lead to bad breath, heartburn, and upset stomach.

Contraindications: Do not take if allergic to garlic or if pregnant or breast-feeding.

Alternatives: All close relatives of onions and garlic including shallots, leeks, chive, and rakkyo.

Other Uses: Blood pressure, digestion, stomach ulcers, cancer, blood clotting, impotence, antiseptic, hair loss, etc.

Garlic, raw		
Nutritional value per 100 g (3.5 oz)		
Energy	623 kJ (149 kcal)	
Carbohydrates	33.06 g	
Sugars	1 g	
Dietary fiber	2.1 g	
Fat	0.5 g	
Protein	6.36 g	
Vitamins	**Quantity**	**%DV**[†]
Thiamine (B$_1$)	0.2 mg	17%
Riboflavin (B$_2$)	0.11 mg	9%
Niacin (B$_3$)	0.7 mg	5%
Pantothenic acid (B$_5$)	0.596 mg	12%
Vitamin B$_6$	1.2350 mg	95%
Folate (B$_9$)	3 µg	1%
Choline	23.2 mg	5%
Vitamin C	31.2 mg	38%
Minerals	**Quantity**	**%DV**[†]
Calcium	181 mg	18%
Iron	1.7 mg	13%
Magnesium	25 mg	7%
Manganese	1.672 mg	80%
Phosphorus	153 mg	22%
Potassium	401 mg	9%
Sodium	17 mg	1%
Zinc	1.16 mg	12%
Other constituents	**Quantity**	
Water	59 g	
selenium	14.2 µg	

2. Honey

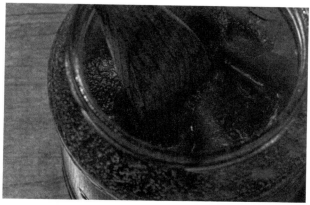

Honey has been applied in Chinese medicine, long before antibiotics were invented elsewhere, as an antibacterial treatment because it contains an antimicrobial enzyme that releases hydrogen peroxide and prevents the growth of specific bacteria. Honey was used in Chinese medicine to relieve pain, neutralize toxins, and harmonize the liver. It has proven especially effective for treating stomach ulcers or the bacterium *Helicobacter pylori*. Did you know that honey never goes bad? It may be kept without preservatives for years.

TIP: Honey is very effective to treat cough, cold, phlegm, and asthma. It is especially very effective when you take a teaspoon with half a teaspoon of black pepper first thing in the morning. Take only for three days at a time.

Availability: In most food-based shops. (e.g. iHerb.com, Amazon.com, herbalremedies.com)

Antibiotic Properties: A high viscosity and enzymatic production of hydrogen peroxide. *Primarily used for treating wounds and burns.* Remember, the darker the honey, the higher the antibiotic quality.

Collection & Preparation: Honey can be consumed in food or used topically on skin. Best used as antiseptic (locally).

Dosage: 15-30 ml per day. Avoid excessive usage.

Possible Side Effects: Could react badly if allergic to pollen.

Contraindications: Infants can contract botulism – a paralytic illness produced by bacteria – from honey.

Alternatives: N/A.

Other Uses: Gastric disturbances, ulcers, wounds, burns, diabetes, allergies, cough, cancer, etc.

Honey

Nutritional value per 100 g (3.5 oz)		
Energy	1,272 kJ (304 kcal)	
Carbohydrates	82.4 g	
Sugars	82.12 g	
Dietary fiber	0.2 g	
Fat	0 g	
Protein	0.3 g	
Vitamins	**Quantity**	**%DV[†]**
Riboflavin (B$_2$)	0.038 mg	3%
Niacin (B$_3$)	0.121 mg	1%
Pantothenic acid (B$_5$)	0.068 mg	1%
Vitamin B$_6$	0.024 mg	2%
Folate (B$_9$)	2 µg	1%
Vitamin C	0.5 mg	1%
Minerals	**Quantity**	**%DV[†]**
Calcium	6 mg	1%
Iron	0.42 mg	3%
Magnesium	2 mg	1%
Phosphorus	4 mg	1%
Potassium	52 mg	1%
Sodium	4 mg	0%
Zinc	0.22 mg	2%
Other constituents	**Quantity**	
Water	17.10 g	

3. Cabbage

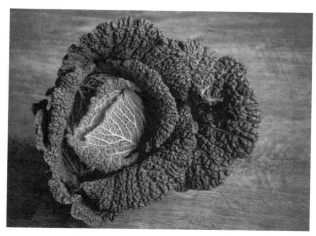

Cabbage is well-known for its healing properties. A major reason is its cancer-fighting sulphur compounds. Additionally, it is well-known that vegetables and fruits high in Vitamin C work as a natural antibiotic. Just one cup of cabbage can provide nearly 75% of an adult's daily allowance of Vitamin C. Cabbage is a member of the Cruciferous family, with vegetables like Brussels sprouts, kale, broccoli, and cauliflower.

TIP: Did you know that stomach ulcers can be treated with fresh cabbage juice? Over the course of two weeks, consume a half-cup of fresh cabbage juice 2-3 times a day between meals. Try adding a half-teaspoon of raw, unfiltered honey, for its pain-relieving properties. Sip slowly and chew the mixture just a bit to move the enzymes around. Additionally, did you know that raw cabbage leaves can relieve inflammation from menstrual breast tenderness, mastitis, and fibro cysts when applied topically to tender breasts?

Availability: In most food-based shops. (e.g. Asda)

Antibiotic Properties: High in glutamine and Vitamin K. *Primarily used for asthma, cancer, and morning sickness.*

Collection & Preparation: Eaten raw or in a juice form is most effective.

Dosage: Include raw cabbage in regular diet every day.

Possible Side Effects: Raised sugar and glucose levels, check with a doctor if you're using any medication. It may also cause blisters. Excessive use may cause constipation.

Contraindications: Diabetics may have their blood sugar affected; people who suffer with an underactive thyroid may have their condition worsened. Avoid during pregnancy or breastfeeding.

Alternatives: Closely related cole crops such as broccoli and cauliflower.

Other Uses: Breast calming, weight loss, acid reflux, candidiasis, cancer, headaches, etc.

Cabbage, raw

Nutritional value per 100 g (3.5 oz)		
Energy	103 kJ (25 kcal)	
Carbohydrates	5.8 g	
Sugars	3.2 g	
Dietary fiber	2.5 g	
Fat	0.1 g	
Protein	1.28 g	
Vitamins	**Quantity**	**%DV†**
Thiamine (B$_1$)	0.061 mg	5%
Riboflavin (B$_2$)	0.040 mg	3%
Niacin (B$_3$)	0.234 mg	2%
Pantothenic acid (B$_5$)	0.212 mg	4%
Vitamin B$_6$	0.124 mg	10%
Folate (B$_9$)	43 µg	11%
Vitamin C	36.6 mg	44%
Vitamin K	76 µg	72%
Minerals	**Quantity**	**%DV†**
Calcium	40 mg	4%
Iron	0.47 mg	4%
Magnesium	12 mg	3%
Manganese	0.16 mg	8%
Phosphorus	26 mg	4%
Potassium	170 mg	4%
Sodium	18 mg	1%
Zinc	0.18 mg	2%
Other constituents	**Quantity**	
Fluoride	1 µg	

4. Calendula (Marigold)

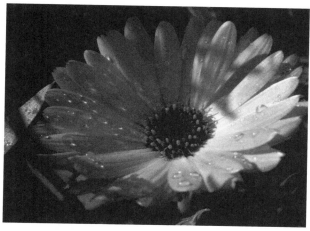

The *Calendula officinalis* flower petals have been applied since at least the twelfth century as medicine in Ancient Greece, Rome, and Indian cultures. Many plant-oriented pharmacological studies suggest that extracts of calendula may provide anti-inflammatory, antiviral, and anti-genotoxic properties in vitro. One study showed that the methanol calendula extract displayed antibacterial activity, where the ethanol and methanol extracts displayed antifungal activities. The pot marigold and horsetails are just a couple of the plants considered astringent without a high concentration of tannins.

TIP: Calendula is available in the form of a tincture at homeopathic pharmacies, and it's called Marigold Tincture. Always keep a bottle at home because it's excellent for bleeding cuts. Dress the wound with the tincture diluted with water (half and half) and bandage.

Availability: In most good herbal remedy stores. (e.g. iHerb.com, Amazon.com, mountainroseherbs.com)

Antibiotic Properties: Faradiol-3-O-palmitate, faradiol-3-O-myristate, faradiol-3-O-laurate, arnidiol-3-O-palmitate, arnidiol-3-O-myristate, arnidiol-3-O-laurate, calenduladiol-3-O-palmitate, and calenduladiol-3-O-myristate. *Primarily used for menstrual pain, aphthous ulcers and the cream focuses on skin issues.*

Collection & Preparation: Petals must be dried out over 4-6 weeks. Can be bought as a tonic, a cream or prepared in food.

Dosage: 2-3 cups of infusion daily. Steep 5-10 g (1 tsp) of dried calendula florets in 250 ml (8 oz) of water for 10-15 minutes.

Possible Side Effects: Do not use if allergic to ragweed; drowsiness can be caused.

Contraindications: Can affect conception. Also do not use when on sedatives, blood pressure medication, or diabetes medication. Avoid while nursing, and taking calendula internally during pregnancy may cause miscarriage.

Alternatives: N/A.

Other Uses: Burns, wounds, blepharitis, dermatitis, ear infections, bruises, acne, etc.

5. Cinnamon

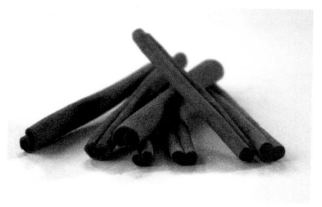

A group of surgeons conducted research that found a cinnamon oil solution could fight common infections, many of which originated in hospitals. MRSA and streptococcus are just two of those hospital-acquired infections. Cinnamon oil could be as effective as the antiseptics used to fight infections that are caused by these bacteria, and the oil could be applied directly in those originating hospitals. Another study, from French scientists, discovered that cinnamon oil with 10% strength or less could combat a variety of bacteria strains, such as E.coli and staphylococcus, which are resistant to traditional antibiotics.

Cinnamon can be combined with honey to fight a variety of infections. Using these two products daily can help prevent viral and bacterial infections because they can strengthen white blood cells. Drink them with water to heal bladder infections and coughs and colds. A paste made from cinnamon and honey can cure acne, eczema, and other skin infections; ease a toothache, insect bites, and ringworm.

TIP: Did you know that chewing cinnamon sticks daily is a very effective way to treat gout?

Availability: In most good health food and herbal remedy stores. (e.g. iHerb.com, Amazon.com, healthspan.co.uk)

Antibiotic Properties: Cinnamaldehyde, cinnamyl acetate, and cinnamyl alcohol. Cinnamon strengthens white blood cells and helps the body to fight off infections. *Primarily used for diabetes symptoms and indigestion.*

Collection & Preparation: Can be taken as juice, powder or prepared with food. Also can be bought as tablets and capsules.

Dosage: 1-6 g per day for no longer than six weeks.

Possible Side Effects: Increased heart rate and palpitations.

Contraindications: Do not take if using blood-thinners such as Warfarin. Also avoid it if you experience prostate problems.

Alternatives: N/A.

Other Uses: Improving glucose and lipid levels, gout, high blood pressure, HIV, multiple sclerosis, etc.

6. Clove

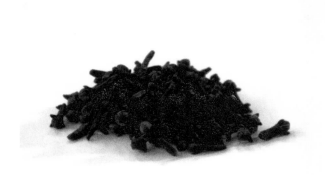

Cloves are widely recognized the world over for their culinary and medicinal properties. This spice belongs to the Myrtaceae family, and cloves are the "flower buds" from an Indonesian evergreen rain-forest tree. The buds begin pale in color but develop their well-known bright-red hue by harvesting time. They are typically picked when they reach nearly 2 cm in length.

TIP: Clove is very effective in helping you to avoid premature ejaculation. For a few days, apply a few drops of clove oil topically with a carrier oil, such as sesame oil, by massaging the penis with it for around 15 minutes per day.

Availability: In most good health food and herbal remedy stores. (e.g. store.newwayherbs.com, iHerb.com)

Antibiotic Properties: Eugenol. Brilliant for digestive and respiratory support, boosting your immune system, and eliminating bad breath or aphthous ulcers. Clove oil is *primarily used to numb and relieve pain*. It's very effective to relieve toothache.

Collection & Preparation: Buy whole cloves rather than powder, store them in a cool, dark place, and cook them within your food. Also available as an oil or essential oil.

Dosage: For toothache, gargle a cup of warm water, with 2-3 drops of clove oil added, 3-4 times daily. For bloating, drink one glass of water daily with 4-5 drops of clove oil added.

Possible Side Effects: Dermatitis, vomiting, dizziness, diarrhea, and bloating.

Contraindications: Do not use if allergic to eugenol, suffer from Crohn's disease, or have liver problems. Avoid use of cloves and clove oil during pregnancy. Can also cause irritation if used in its pure form.

Alternatives: Basil, marjoram, cinnamon.

Other Uses: Digestion issues, lack of appetite, travel sickness, respiration diseases, acid reflux, candidiasis, etc.

7. Echinacea

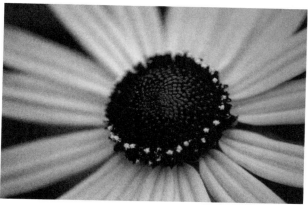

Echinacea has been used as an herbal remedy for over a century. This native American healing plant will boost your immune system, which is its plan of attack against bacteria. Echinacea is still the subject of current research, but there is recorded evidence that it helps your body generate white blood cells, including T-lymphocytes, and release interferon. This infection-fighting protein kills germs by preventing them from replicating. Additionally, Echinacea helps immune-system cells generate more macrophages, or germ-eating cells, and supports the germ-killing process of phagocytosis. This healing herb also supports the immune system by hindering a bacteria's secretion of hyaluronidase, an enzyme that enables the breakdown of a cell's protective membranes, and invasion of tissues, and by seeking out and destroying the flu and common cold viruses.

TIP: Echinacea helps your body create powerful cells that enhance your immune system to combat bacterial infections. Boil 2-3 teaspoons of ground, dried echinacea in a cup of water, then strain. Drink the tea twice daily. Or, make the echinacea infusion, soak a cotton ball in it, then dab directly on the affected area.

Availability: From most good herbal remedy shops. (e.g. avogel.co.uk, iHerb.com, Amazon.com)

Antibiotic Properties: Polysaccharides, glycoproteins, alkamides, volatile oils, and flavonoids. An immunostimulant that helps the body boost its immune system. *Primarily used for upper respiratory tract infections – such as a cold or bacterial infections.*

Collection & Preparation: Can be taken as an herb juice, a tincture, a freeze-dried capsule, or a tablet. You can also make a tea by drying the roots out for two weeks and brewing them with 8 oz of water.

Dosage: Juice 6-9 ml for three weeks, capsule 100 mg three times a day, tablet 6.78 mg three times a day. A tincture is the most recommended method for consuming it. Avoid using for longer than 3 weeks.

Possible Side Effects: Itchiness or a rash. High doses of echinacea may cause nausea, dizziness, insomnia, or headaches.

Contraindications: Do not take if pregnant, suffering with autoimmune disorders, such as MS, or allergic to ragweed. Also check with your doctor for possible interaction with other medicine, e.g. heart medication, antifungal or anti-anxiety drugs.

Alternatives: N/A.

Other Uses: Influenza, urinary tract infections, vaginal yeast infections, genital herpes, gum disease, acne, psoriasis, sinus infections, candidiasis, asthma, etc.

8. Oregon Grape Root

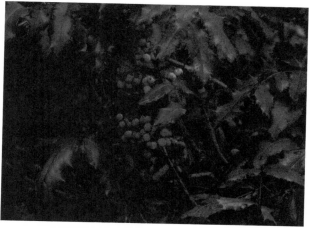

Oregon grape, like goldenseal, contains berberine, which has been proven to offer antiseptic protection from fungus, bacteria, and viruses by scientific research. Because Oregon grape root has a soothing effect on the smooth muscles of the digestive tract, herbalists will apply it to treat intestinal parasites, stomach cramps, bacterial diarrhea, and abdominal pain – in addition to eye infection and plaque psoriasis. The advantage to applying mixtures with the whole herb, versus products with berberine extracts, is Oregon grape root's tannins, which can ease itchy skin, irritation, and inflammation. Due to their having berberine in common, Oregon grape root can serve as a goldenseal substitute.

Availability: Available in most good herbal remedy shops. (e.g. <u>iHerb.com</u>)

Antibiotic Properties: Berberine. Oregon grape root works well alongside conventional medicine as it is thought to give antibiotics 'in' to the right cells. *Primarily used for liver and eye problems.*

Collection & Preparation: Available as a cream or capsules. Can also be made into a tea by simmering 1-2 teaspoons of coarsely cut root for 10-15 minutes.

Dosage: Take for no longer than a week, leaving at least a seven-day break.

Possible Side Effects: Can cause jaundice and kernicterus in children.

Contraindications: Do not take while pregnant or suffering from diarrhea.

Alternatives: Barberry, coptis, goldenseal.

Other Uses: Stomach ulcers, psoriasis, acid reflux, dysentery, syphilis, etc.

9. Marshmallow Root

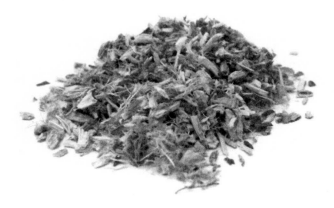

Marshmallow root has many health benefits being a demulcent herb, which means that it is soothing and cooling. Often, it is applied in an effort to enhance digestion and improve hair or skin. Marshmallow root is known as a mucilage, which means it creates a sticky compound that will coat membranes. Note that if a tea is being made with marshmallow root, it needs to be brewed with cold water. This will preserve its mucilaginous properties. It is this aspect that makes marshmallow root effective on inflammatory digestive disorders, because the mucilage remains intact until it is broken down by the colon. Additionally, flavonoids can be found in marshmallow extract, and they work as an anti-inflammatory. The flavonoids reduce inflammation because the mucilage will maintain them and prevent excess damage. Marshmallow extracts will also trigger phagocytosis. This is the process where cells overpower solid particles, bacteria, or dead cell tissues to boost the healing process.

TIP: Did you know that marshmallow can help you quit smoking? Drink a common marshmallow tea twice daily, or purchase capsules and take two of them twice daily.

Availability: From most good herbal remedy stores. (e.g. iHerb.com, Amazon.com, naturesremedy.co.uk)

Antibiotic Properties: Phagocytosis and flavonoids. Marshmallow root forms a protective layer over the skin or digestive system to help them heal.

Primarily used for inflammation calming in mucous membranes.

Collection & Preparation: Can be made into a tea, applied topically, or taken as a tablet.

Dosage: 1-2 teaspoons in boiling water, taken 2-3 times a day. Tablets taken 2-3 times daily.

Possible Side Effects: Low blood sugar levels, breathing problems, skin rashes and itching.

Contraindications: Don't use if you suffer from diabetes. Avoid during pregnancy.

Alternatives: N/A.

Other Uses: Dry coughs, ulcers, gangrene, upset stomach lining, constipation, pain, and swelling, etc.

10. Usnea

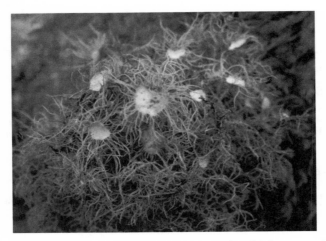

Usnea is a naturally growing herb with antimicrobial properties, which makes it effective against a variety of unwanted pathogens. Therefore, it should not be considered as an antibiotic herb; it doesn't kill bacteria. This is actually good for humans, because the herb is highly effective against a variety of Gram-positive bacteria – for example, strep (*Streptococcus*) and staph (*Staphylococcus simulans* and *S. aureus*) – without disrupting healthy gut microbes. Usnea can also be used to combat diarrhea, urinary tract infections, strep throat, upper respiratory tract infections, tuberculosis, and pneumonia.

Availability: From most good herbal remedy stores. (e.g. iHerb.com, Amazon.com)

Antibiotic Properties: Usnic acid. *Primarily used to decrease inflammation and is great for fever control and pain relief.*

Collection & Preparation: Prepare a tincture where the liquid is half pure grain alcohol and half water; consider a ratio of 1 part usnea to 5 parts liquid.

Dosage: Use 2 teaspoons of tincture in warm water 30 minutes before mealtime three times a day. Do not use for more than two weeks.

Possible Side Effects: May cause gastrointestinal disorders or dermatitis if used topically.

Contraindications: Avoid using during pregnancy and breastfeeding.

Alternatives: N/A.

Other Uses: Pneumonia, vaginal infections, sinus infections, mastitis, candidiasis, influenza. It can also be used in mouthwashes, gargles, and lozenges.

11. Uva Ursi

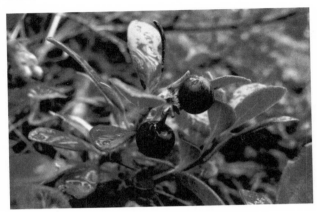

For centuries, uva ursi teas and extracts have been used as a laxative, diuretic, and urinary tract antiseptic. This plant was first documented in a thirteenth-century herbal guide from Wales, but the berries themselves are not used medicinally. This plant's leaves have also been smoked to achieve its benefits. "Bearberry" teas and extracts, because 'uva ursi' translates to "bear's grape" from Latin, have also been used in pharmaceutical preparations. Especially homeopathy, where a leaf tincture is thought to be effective in treating urinary tract inflammations, urethritis, and cystitis.

TIP: Uva ursi promotes the healthy functioning of the kidneys, but aggravates an existing kidney disease. Therefore, do not take uva ursi if you suffer from any kidney problem.

Availability: In most good health food and herbal remedy stores. (e.g. iHerb.com, puritan.com)

Antibiotic Properties: Hydrolysable, ellagic, and gallic acid tannins. There is a sugary molecule in uva ursi that transforms into a natural antibiotic when it gets into your urinary tract. *Primarily used for urinary tract infections.*

Collection & Preparation: Available as tablets, capsules, in crushed leaf or powder forms. Also can be made into a tea by soaking 3 g of dried leaves in 4 oz of water for 12 hours.

Dosage: 400-840 mg daily. Drink a tea 3-4 times daily.

Possible Side Effects: Nausea, vomiting, stomach upset, ringing in your ears.

Contraindications: Do not use if you suffer with retina thinning. Avoid during pregnancy or breastfeeding. Not recommended for children under 12. Avoid if kidney disease exists.

Alternatives: N/A.

Other Uses: Kidney and bladder infections, urinary tract infections, bronchitis, bloating, etc.

12. Yarrow

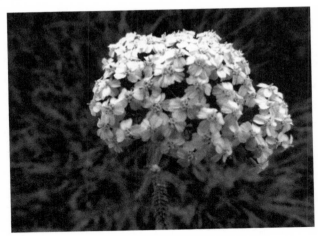

Yarrow, or common yarrow, has been known as *herbal militaris* for its ability to hinder blood flow from open wounds. This flowering plant is a member of the Asteraceae family and native to temperate regions of Asia, North America, and Europe. Yarrow is also known as gordaldo, plumajillo ('little feather' in Spanish), thousand-seal, thousand-leaf, nosebleed plant, soldier's woundwort, old man's pepper, milfoil, devil's nettle, and sanguinary.

TIP: While dried and powered yarrow leaves is one of the best immediate, within seconds, remedies for a nosebleed, fresh sprigs inserted directly into a nostril can make a person's nose bleed.

Availability: In most good herbal remedy stores. (e.g. <u>iHerb.com</u>, <u>discount-supplements.co.uk</u>)

Antibiotic Properties: *Achillea millefolium*. Yarrow increases saliva and stomach acid so it is *primarily used to aid digestion*. It is also super effective for bleeding (internal and external).

Collection & Preparation: It's available as a dried or fresh herb (which can be used in food), a capsule or tablet and liquid extracts or essential oils.

Dosage: No more than 4.5 g per day.

Possible Side Effects: Drowsiness, dermatitis. Long-term use can cause photo-sensitivity to light and headache.

Contraindications: Do not use if you have allergies to plants found in the aster family or when you use high blood pressure or blood-thinning medications or lithium. Avoid use if pregnant or breastfeeding.

Alternatives: N/A.

Other Uses: Loss of appetite, diarrhea, reduce bleeding, fever, menstrual cramps, muscle spasms, TB, etc. Children, people lacking muscular tone, the elderly, and women with anemia are the best people who see yarrow's benefits.

13. Astragalus Root

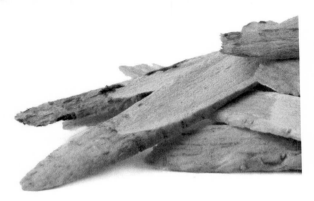

Astragalus is said to provide various benefits for multiple health conditions, such as heart conditions. Its main benefits are stimulating the immune system and inhibiting free radical production with its antioxidant effects. Astragalus comes from a legume or bean and goes by the names *milk vetch* or *huang qi*. There are multiple astragalus species, but most of these herbal supplements contain *astragalus membranaceus*.

TIP: Are you suffering from liver problems? Astragalus is used as a general tonic to protect the liver – it may cure all liver-related problems, including chronic hepatitis.

Availability: Most good herbal remedy stores. (e.g. iHerb.com, Amazon.com, naturesremedy.co.uk)

Antibiotic Properties: Polysaccharides, choline, betaine, rumatakenin, [beta]-sitosterol. Traditional Chinese medicine has made use of the astragalus herb for years because it's an adaptogen, which means that it's great for helping the body against physical, mental, and emotional stress. *It is primarily used for upper respiratory infections.*

Collection & Preparation: It is available as a tablet, capsule, powder, or tincture. The root needs to be dried. Can also be made into a tea by mixing 3-6 oz of dried root in 12 oz of water.

Dosage: 200 mg of powder twice a day. Tea can be consumed three times daily. Tincture can be taken three times a day – mix 10-15 drops of tincture in half glass of water.

Possible Side Effects: Can make your immune system more active, so will have an impact on those who suffer from an autoimmune disease.

Contraindications: Do not use if pregnant or breastfeeding; also avoid if you suffer from blood disorders.

Alternatives: N/A.

Other Uses: Dietary supplements, colds, arthritis, asthma, cancer, HIV, AIDS, energy levels, diarrhea, etc.

14. Cat's Claw

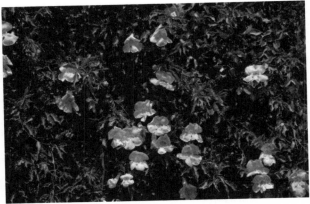

Too few know enough about such a miraculous yet inexpensive Peruvian herb. Cat's claw, *Uncaria tomentosa* or *una de gato*, provides immune-boosting properties from oxindole alkaloids found in the plant's bark and roots. Oxindole alkaloids boost white blood cells and their ability to destroy pathogens. Traditionally, for centuries, Peruvian medicine men have applied cat's claw in the treatment of various ailments. This rain-forest vine got its name from the hooked thorns on its twigs, which resemble a cat's claws.

TIP: Cat's claw is best used for stomachache, but it is also used in treating all types of cancer.

Availability: Most good herbal remedy stores. (e.g. iHerb.com, Amazon.com)

Antibiotic Properties: Oxindole alkaloids, which make cat's claw effective in protecting the body's immune system. Cat's claw is *primarily used for arthritis and to fight cold symptoms*.

Collection & Preparation: It is available as a capsule, tincture, or tea – by crushing the vines and mixing them with boiling water.

Dosage: 60-100 mg per day of extract. 20-50 drops of tincture up to three times a day.

Possible Side Effects: Headaches, dizziness, and vomiting. Can cause diarrhea if taken in excess.

Contraindications: Do not take if you suffer from low blood pressure, leukemia, or autoimmune diseases. Also avoid taking during pregnancy or breastfeeding.

Alternatives: N/A.

Other Uses: Bronchitis, asthma, digestive problems, cancer, colitis, anti-inflammatory, fungal issues, Crohn's disease, allergies, etc.

15. Cranberry

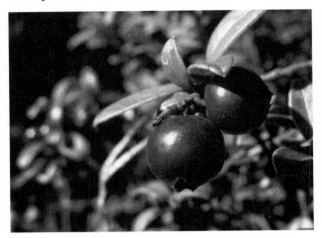

Cranberries contain numerous chemical substances offering beneficial properties, for example, phytonutrients, which are naturally derived plant compounds. Specifically, cranberries contain proanthocyanidin antioxidants, which are important to general wellness and can offer protection from inflammatory diseases, urinary tract infection, and cavities. This berry belongs to the Ericaceae family and is often described as a creeping shrub, an evergreen dwarf, or a low-lying railing vine.

TIP: Did you know that cranberries can combat oral problems like gingivitis and cavities? It prevents food and bacteria from sticking to the teeth. Take 2-3 tablespoons of cranberry juice and swish it in your mouth. Do it daily to prevent bacterial infections.

Availability: In most good health food and herbal remedy stores. (e.g. iHerb.com, Amazon.com, vitabiotics.com)

Antibiotic Properties: Phenolic acids, proanthocyandins, flavonoids. Cranberries create a barrier to protect the urinary tract and is *primarily used for urinary tract infections*.

Collection & Preparation: Can be a juice, or the berries can be included in your diet. You can also buy capsules or tablets to be taken 2-3 times daily.

Dosage: 250 ml of juice twice a day. Avoid excessive consumption.

Possible Side Effects: If you are prone to kidney stones, this possibility can be increased. Excess use may cause diarrhea.

Contraindications: Do not use if you're taking Warfarin – a blood-thinning drug.

Alternatives: Barley or wheat grass juice.

Other Uses: Antioxidant, urinary tract infections, peptic ulcer, painful ejaculation, cardiovascular disease, gum problems, etc.

Cranberries, raw (*Vaccinium macrocarpon*)

Nutritional value per 100 g (3.5 oz)		
Energy	46 kcal (190 kJ)	
Carbohydrates	12.2 g	
Sugars	4.04 g	
Dietary fiber	4.6 g	
Fat	0.13 g	
Protein	0.39 g	
Vitamins	**Quantity**	**%DV†**
Vitamin A equiv.	3 µg	0%
beta-Carotene	36 µg	0%
lutein zeaxanthin	91 µg	
Thiamine (B$_1$)	0.012 mg	1%
Riboflavin (B$_2$)	0.02 mg	2%
Niacin (B$_3$)	0.101 mg	1%
Pantothenic acid (B$_5$)	0.295 mg	6%
Vitamin B$_6$	0.057 mg	4%
Folate (B$_9$)	1 µg	0%
Vitamin C	13.3 mg	16%
Vitamin E	1.2 mg	8%
Vitamin K	5.1 µg	5%
Minerals	**Quantity**	**%DV†**
Calcium	8 mg	1%
Iron	0.25 mg	2%
Magnesium	6 mg	2%
Manganese	0.36 mg	17%
Phosphorus	13 mg	2%
Potassium	85 mg	2%
Sodium	2 mg	0%
Zinc	0.1 mg	1%
Other constituents	**Quantity**	
Water	87.13 g	

16. Elderberry

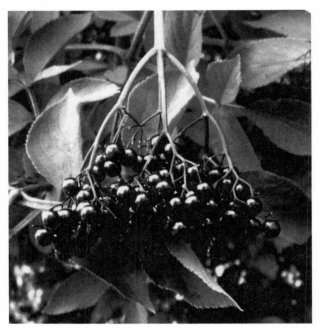

For centuries, elderberries have been used as a folk remedy in North Africa, Western Asia, North America, and Europe. Recognized for their antioxidant properties, elderberries have been applied as a diaphoretic, diuretic, and laxative, while also being used to boost the immune system; alleviate coughs, flu, colds, tonsillitis, viral and bacterial infections; improve vision, lower cholesterol, and improve heart health. In 1995, a flu epidemic in Panama was treated with elderberry juice. Which explains why the medicinal benefits of these berries are currently being rediscovered and investigated.

Elderberries contain flavonoids, viburnic acid, and Vitamins A, B, and C. Elderberry's therapeutic properties, found in the flowers and berries, are believed to be drawn from their flavonoids. Which, according to research, include anthocyanins that protect cells against damage and act as powerful antioxidants.

Availability: In most good health food and herbal remedy stores. (e.g. iHerb.com, Amazon.com, lewtress.co.uk)

Antibiotic Properties: Carotenoids, flavonoids, anthocyanins. Elderberries reduce the swelling in the mucous membranes, so they're *primarily used for sinus infections.*

Collection & Preparation: Can be taken as a juice or used in your food.

You can also buy elderberry liquid capsules.

Dosage: Take the juice extracts for no longer than twelve weeks or 15 ml four times a day. Do not let up on the dosage, as the elderberry must stay consistently in the body for it to do its job.

Possible Side Effects: Nausea, vomiting, and severe diarrhea. Can decrease blood sugar.

Contraindications: Do not use if you suffer from autoimmune diseases or take immune system suppressants. Do not take if you use laxatives.

Alternatives: N/A.

Other Uses: Reduces cancer cell formation, antioxidant, protects blood vessels, effective for bleeding, flu, facial neuralgia, rheumatoid arthritis, etc.

Elderberries, raw
Sambucus spp.

Nutritional value per 100 g (3.5 oz)		
Energy	305 kJ (73 kcal)	
Carbohydrates	18.4 g	
Dietary fiber	7 g	
Fat	0.5 g	
Protein	0.66 g	
Vitamins	**Quantity**	**%DV†**
Vitamin A equiv.	30 µg	4%
Thiamine (B$_1$)	0.07 mg	6%
Riboflavin (B$_2$)	0.06 mg	5%
Niacin (B$_3$)	0.5 mg	3%
Pantothenic acid (B$_5$)	0.14 mg	3%
Vitamin B$_6$	0.23 mg	18%
Folate (B$_9$)	6 µg	2%
Vitamin C	36 mg	43%
Minerals	**Quantity**	**%DV†**
Calcium	38 mg	4%
Iron	1.6 mg	12%
Magnesium	5 mg	1%
Phosphorus	39 mg	6%
Potassium	280 mg	6%
Zinc	0.11 mg	1%
Other constituents	**Quantity**	
Water	79.80 g	

17. Ginger

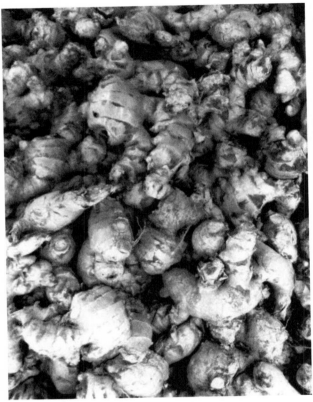

Ginger, or *Zingiber officinale,* has seen medicinal use for the last 2,000 years, at least, on top of its culinary properties, which may stem from its well-known capability soothe digestion or gastrointestinal issues, including acid reflux and ulcerative colitis. However, ginger has also proven more effective than antibiotics in fighting bacterial staph infections. This plant has effective anti-inflammatory properties, alleviating brain inflammations specifically, and has destroyed cancer cells. Ginger can even boost the immune system and alleviate gamma radiation effects. Some of the chemical components that support ginger's health benefits are gingerols (providing pain-relief properties), zingerone, and shogaol. Both medicinal and culinary properties are found in the rhizomes, which are the root-looking stems of the plant that grow under the ground.

TIP: Did you know that ginger can alleviate hay fever? Boil 2-3 small ginger pieces with a cup of water for 5-6 minutes, then strain well. Mix in some raw honey. Consume 2-3 times daily for two weeks.

Availability: In most good health food and herbal remedy stores. (e.g. iHerb.com, Amazon.com, naturesbest.co.uk)

Antibiotic Properties: Rhizome. Ginger provides anti-inflammatory properties, which means that it *primarily used as a pain reliever.*

Collection & Preparation: Can be bought as food, drink, sweets, powder, capsules, tinctures, and tablets. Ginger can be made into a tea by mixing a tablespoon of fresh grated ginger with boiling water.

Dosage: Capsules or tablets – 250 mg four times a day. Avoid excessive consumption.

Possible Side Effects: Heartburn, stomach discomfort, extra menstrual bleeding, irritation. When taken in large dosages, can cause high blood pressure.

Contraindications: Do not take if using Warfarin, diabetes medication, heart medication, or aspirin. Avoid ginger oil during pregnancy.

Alternatives: Honey.

Other Uses: Hay fever, allergies, nausea, vomiting, cancer, diabetics, ulcers, gastric distress, inflammation, radiation, high blood pressure, arthritis, angina, etc.

Ginger root (raw)

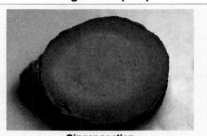

Ginger section

Nutritional value per 100 g (3.5 oz)

Energy	333 kJ (80 kcal)
Carbohydrates	17.77 g
Sugars	1.7 g
Dietary fiber	2 g
Fat	0.75 g
Protein	1.82 g

Vitamins	**Quantity**	**%DV**[†]
Thiamine (B$_1$)	0.025 mg	2%
Riboflavin (B$_2$)	0.034 mg	3%
Niacin (B$_3$)	0.75 mg	5%
Pantothenic acid (B$_5$)	0.203 mg	4%
Vitamin B$_6$	0.16 mg	12%
Folate (B$_9$)	11 µg	3%
Vitamin C	5 mg	6%
Vitamin E	0.26 mg	2%

Minerals	**Quantity**	**%DV**[†]
Calcium	16 mg	2%
Iron	0.6 mg	5%
Magnesium	43 mg	12%
Manganese	0.229 mg	11%
Phosphorus	34 mg	5%
Potassium	415 mg	9%
Sodium	13 mg	1%
Zinc	0.34 mg	4%

Other constituents	**Quantity**
Water	79 g

18. Lemon Balm

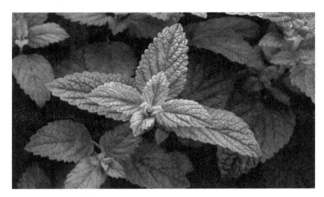

Lemon balm, or *Melissa officinalis*, has a centuries-long history of being used to improve digestion, enhance sleep, and alleviate anxiety. Upon research, experts have found this calming herb provides several other health benefits. It was used by the ancient Romans and Greeks to treat insect stings and bites. The leaves give off a tart, lemon-like aroma that will also repel insects because they contain monoterpene aldehydes citral A and B and citronella. Lemon balm is a member of the mint family and can be grown anywhere in the world. Often, it is included in gardens to attract bees and boost pollination. It can get as tall as two feet and sprouts yellow flowers.

TIP: Did you know that lemon balm cures herpes? Make leaf decoction of lemon balm and apply it over canker sores using a cotton ball.

Availability: In most good herbal remedy and health food stores. (e.g. iHerb.com, Amazon.com, naturesremedy.co.uk)

Antibiotic Properties: Citral, citronella, flavonoids. Lemon balm has been proven to reduce stress in the central nervous system, which means it is *primarily used for dementia and Alzheimer's disease.*

Collection & Preparation: Available as a capsule or can be made into a tea by mixing 1 oz of fresh lemon balm leaves with boiling water. Also available as essential oil or tincture.

Dosage: 80 mg per day of powder (capsules), or 50-60 drops of tincture in water for no longer than four months. Can be taken as infusion of dried herb or fresh leaves (4-6 leaves). Drink twice a day.

Possible Side Effects: Abdominal pain, dizziness, wheezing, drowsiness.

Contraindications: Do not allow children under the age of 12 to take. Always consult a doctor before using it.

Alternatives: N/A.

Other Uses: Anxiety, sleep problems, stomach disorders, anemia, restless-ness, high blood pressure, insect bites, etc.

19. Licorice Root

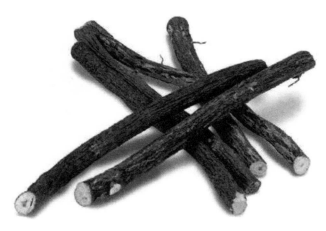

Licorice root is well-known as an herbal medicine with a lengthy list of beneficial uses; despite that, it is still considered one of the most over-looked herbal remedies available. It is often applied as a substitute for St. John's wort and contains antidepressant compounds. This powerful root is applied in the treatment of many ailments, such as arthritis, asthma, prostate enlargement, athlete's foot, yeast infections, baldness, ulcers, body odor, tuberculosis, bursitis, tendinitis, canker sores, sore throat, chronic fatigue, shingles, depression, psoriasis, colds and flu, menopause, coughs, Lyme disease, dandruff, liver problems, emphysema, fungal infections, gingivitis and tooth decay, viral infections, gout, HIV, and heartburn.

TIP: Did you know that licorice candy typically contains anise oil?

Availability: Most good herbal remedy and health food shops. (e.g. <u>Amazon.com</u>, <u>hollandandbarrett.com</u>)

Antibiotic Properties: Glycyrrhizin, which heals the mucous membranes of the digestive tract, making it great for healing the gastrointestinal system. Licorice root is *primarily used for stomach inflammation.*

Collection & Preparation: Can be prepared in food or bought in medicinal tincture form, powder, or capsules.

Dosage: Make a tea with 2 ml of powdered root mixed with a cup of water, then boil and let it simmer for 10 minutes. Consume three times daily. Avoid using for more than 6 weeks.

Possible Side Effects: High blood pressure, low potassium levels, fatigue, water and sodium retention. Edema, dizziness, may reduce libido.

Contraindications: Do not use if you suffer from high blood pressure, diabetes, hormone sensitive conditions, kidney disease, hypertonia, heart disease or are pregnant or breastfeeding.

Alternatives: St. John's wort.

Other Uses: Cough, bronchitis, colitis, lower cholesterol, ulcers, skin disorders, liver problems, asthma, etc.

20. Mullein

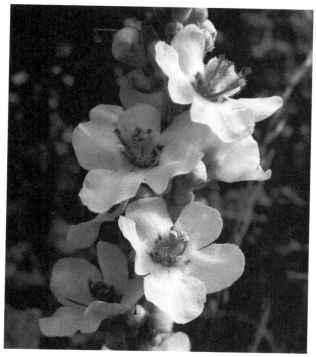

Mullein, *Verbascum thapsus*, is frequently used in herbal medicine for its gastrointestinal benefits. Mullein, or "mullein leaf," comprises about 250 species of flowering plants in the Scrophulariaceae family, which are native to Asia and Europe.

TIP: Did you know that mullein is very effective in getting rid of intestinal worms and other gastrointestinal issues?

Availability: Most good herbal remedy and health food shops. (e.g. iHerb.com, Amazon.com)

Antibiotic Properties: Verbascoside. Mullein's mucilage and saponins ensures that it is a great herb for respiratory infections. It's *primarily used for bleeding and fever symptoms.*

Collection & Preparation: Often served as medicinal tea. Can be bought as a capsule or tincture.

Dosage: Combine half a teaspoon of powdered leaves or root in a cup of water, then boil and let it simmer it for 10 minutes. Consume three times a day. One teaspoon of tincture can be taken two times a day for 10-14 days.

Possible Side Effects: Skin irritation, breathing difficulties, stomach pain.

Contraindications: Avoid using while pregnant or breastfeeding.

Alternatives: N/A.

Other Uses: Whooping cough, tuberculosis, bronchitis, asthma, joint pain, gout, ear trouble, skin problems, etc.

21. Olive Leaf

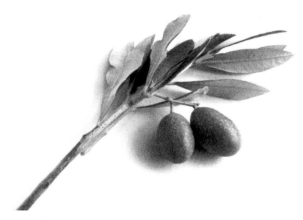

The olive tree (*Olea europaea*) contains a unique molecule, known as *oleuropein*, that provides its multitude of life-extending and medicinal benefits. Oleuropein is a polyphenol that provides olive oil's disease-fighting, anti-inflammatory, and antioxidant properties and helps lower blood pressure and bad cholesterol, protect against cognitive decline, guard against oxidative damage, and prevent cancer. In one study, when the polyphenol was administered to animals with tumors, those growths were repressed and disappeared in 9-12 days. However, recent research has determined that oleuropein's benefits may reach well beyond that, showing promise in combatting diabetes, atherosclerosis, neurodegenerative diseases, cancer, and arthritis. Oleuropein, which grows in the tree's leaves and fruit, is the origin of that distinctive pungent, tangy, nearly bitter flavor high-quality extra virgin olive oils are known for. New specialized extraction techniques support the collection of a standardized and more stable strain of oleuropein.

TIP: Did you know that you can use olive oil for snoring? Simply put 1 drop of olive oil in both nostrils before going to bed. To lower cholesterol levels, take one or two teaspoons of olive oil daily.

Availability: Most good herbal remedy and health food shops. (e.g. iHerb.com, Amazon.com)

Antibiotic Properties: Oleuropein, which breaks down the cell walls of pathogen bacteria. Olive leaves are *primarily used for lowering blood pressure and cholesterol.*

Collection & Preparation: Can be consumed with food (olive oil) or purchased as a liquid extract.

Dosage: Liquid extract 30 ml per day or with food 30-40 g.

Possible Side Effects: Can affect respiration allergies or cause allergic reactions if applying on skin.

Contraindications: Do not use if pregnant, breastfeeding or suffer from diabetes.

Alternatives: N/A.

Other Uses: High blood pressure, oral herpes, eczema, measles, insect bites, cancer, age-related diseases, arthritis, etc.

22. Oregano

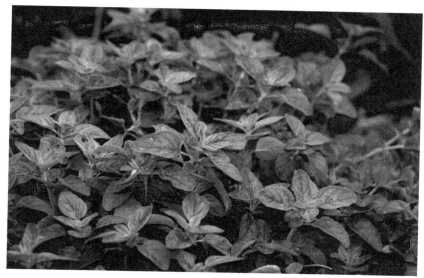

Oregano oil, distilled from the plant's flowers and leaves, can be used in various ways to defend the body against bacterial infections. This oil contains *carvacrol*, a compound that can help break through the cell membranes that protect bacteria from a body's immune system. Because of this, oregano oil has been proven an effective bacteria killer that boosts the immune system to take better action against parasites, fungi, and viruses.

TIP: Did you know that oregano contains 42 times more antioxidants than an apple? It is great anti-aging food. Also, if you suffer from menstrual cramps, try chewing 4-5 fresh leaves of oregano to alleviate the cramping.

Availability: Most good herbal remedy and health food shops. (e.g. iHerb.com, Amazon.com, puritan.com)

Antibiotic Properties: Carvacrol and thymol, which help kill bacteria by breaking through the cell membranes that protect them. Oregano is *primarily used for respiratory tract infections and candidiasis.*

Collection & Preparation: It can be used in food or bought as oil and capsules.

Dosage: Use one part of oregano oil diluted with two parts of olive oil for external uses. For internal use, mix a cup of water with 2-3 drops of oregano oil.

Possible Side Effects: Can cause a reaction if you're allergic to plants in the Lamiaceae family. It may also cause skin irritation and stomach upset.

Contraindications: Do not take if you suffer from bleeding disorders or diabetes. Avoid use during pregnancy and while breastfeeding.

Alternatives: N/A.

Other Uses: Muscle pain, athlete's foot, dandruff, wrinkles, asthma, cuts and bruises, earaches, influenza, acne, varicose veins, etc.

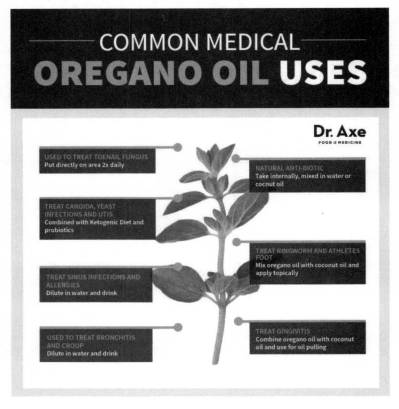

23. Black Seed

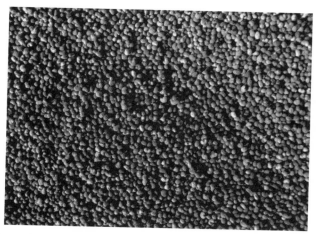

Black seed, or *Nigella sativa*, has gone by many names throughout its long history of use as a healing herb: onion seed, Roman coriander, black cumin, and black sesame. The earliest record of black seed's use and cultivation comes from ancient Egypt, approximately 3,300 years ago, when black seed oil was recovered from Pharaoh Tutankhamun's tomb. Among Arabic cultures, black seed, referred to as black cumin, has been known as *Habbatul barakah*, which translates to "seed of blessing." There is also a myth that Mohammed, the Islamic prophet, said black cumin is "a remedy for all diseases except death."

TIP: Did you know that black cumin seeds are healthy for women? It helps with proper menstruation and also enhances milk flow in lactating mothers. It is also advisable to use it immediately after a delivery because it helps to clean the uterus.

Availability: In most good herbal remedy and health food shops. (e.g. iHerb.com, Amazon.com, amazingherbs.com)

Antibiotic Properties: Thymoquinone, thymohydroquinone, dithymoquinone, thymol, carvacrol, nigellicine, and alpha-hederin – all of which work towards boosting your immune system. Black seed is mostly known for its work in *HIV treatment*. It is also used for *pain relief.*

Collection & Preparation: Mix the oil with another liquid, such as juice or yogurt. The seeds must be heated. It is also available as a powder.

Dosage: 3 teaspoons per day.

Possible Side Effects: Do not take if pregnant – black seed can prevent the uterus from contracting.

Contraindications: Do not take if you suffer from bleeding disorders, diabetes, or low blood pressure. Consult a doctor before consuming.

Alternatives: N/A.

Other Uses: Sore throat, headaches, asthma, hay fever, bronchitis, constipation, combating the side effects of chemotherapy, etc.

24. Acacia (Catechu)

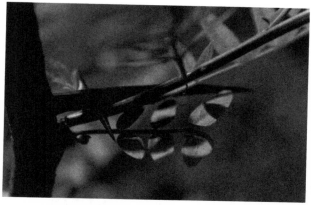

Acacia has currently become popular because herbalists are recommending it as a natural remedy, based on its therapeutic properties, for various disorders. For thousands of years, these trees have been sought out for their medicinal properties, strong wood, and decorative uses. There is even a legend, among Hebrews who consider it to be sacred, that Jesus's crown of thorns was made from acacia.

TIP: Did you know that acacia can help you with obesity? Simply powder it, take a pinch, and mix it in one glass of lukewarm water. Drink twice a day for seven days. Do not use it for more than seven days.

Availability: In most good herbal remedy stores. (e.g. <u>iHerb.com</u>, <u>Amazon.com</u>, <u>puritan.com</u>)

Antibiotic Properties: Staphylococcus and tusca, which works as a fiber – aiding the digestive system. Acacia is *primarily known for lowering cholesterol.*

Collection & Preparation: Available as seeds, powder, honey, and a gum that needs to be combined with water to work successfully.

Dosage: 30 g of powder daily for six weeks.

Possible Side Effects: Gas, bloating, nausea and loose stools, hypotension.

Contraindications: Avoid use when pregnant or breastfeeding.

Alternatives: N/A.

Other Uses: Weight loss aid, throat and stomach inflammation, skin diseases, eyes bloodshot, anemia, etc.

For 7 uses of Acacia go to <u>healthline.com/health/7-uses-for-acacia</u>

25. Aloe

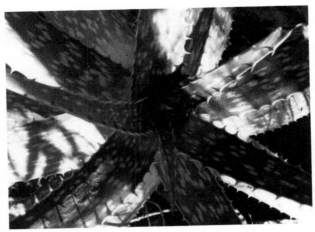

Aloe vera (commonly called *Aloe*) is known for its medicinal properties, and the plant produces *gel* and *latex* substances that are both therapeutic. The gel is a clear, jelly-like product extracted from the inner part of the leaf. Latex is a yellow product extracted from under the plant's skin. There are aloe products that can be made from the whole leaf, which means they contain both latex and gel.

TIP: Aloe vera contains aloin, which eases the effects of hangover. It reduces problems like dry mouth, dehydration, and headache. It also relaxes the nerves and prevents the conversion of alcohol into harmful substances.

Availability: In most good herbal remedy stores. (e.g. puritan.com, iHerb.com, Amazon.com)

Antibiotic Properties: Vitamin B12, phenolic compounds, saponins, amino acids, anthraquinones, sterols, and salicylic acid. These have a keratolytic effect on wounds – which helps remove dead tissue. It's *primarily used for skin issues*.

Collection & Preparation: Available in various forms – gel, latex, cream, or drinks.

Dosage: 100-200 mg gel, 50 mg aloe latex, or 0.5 g cream applied three times a day.

Possible Side Effects: Aloe latex can cause stomach cramps, low potassium, kidney problems, blood in urine, and heart disturbances. It may also cause skin allergy.

Contraindications: Do not take if under 12 years old, suffer from Crohn's disease, kidney or bowel problems, or hemorrhoids. Avoid consuming Aloe vera juice if pregnant.

Alternatives: N/A.

Other Uses: Burns, immune system boost, scars, ulcers, diabetes, cancer, hair loss, skin cell rejuvenation, obesity, etc.

26. Cryptolepis

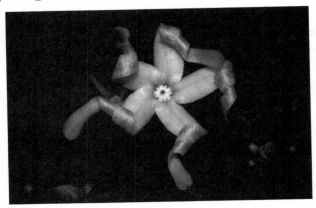

Cryptolepis sanguinolenta is applied as a powerful antibiotic and has the potential to treat Type 2 diabetes. A cryptolepis root extract is typically used to treat malaria in West Africa. This species of flowering plant is in the Apocynaceae family.

Availability: In most good herbal remedy stores. (e.g. <u>Amazon.com</u>)

Antibiotic Properties: Alkaloids, isocryptolepine, quindoline, and neocryptine, which build up the body's immune system and is *primarily used for malaria.*

Collection & Preparation: Available as a powder, capsules, or a tincture.

Dosage: Sprinkle powder on affected area, take 2 capsules twice a day, and use tincture twice daily.

Possible Side Effects: Sickness and nausea.

Contraindications: Avoid use when pregnant or breastfeeding.

Alternatives: N/A.

Other Uses: Gonorrhea, TB, urinary tract infections, insomnia, colic, diarrhea, wounds, etc.

27. Eucalyptus

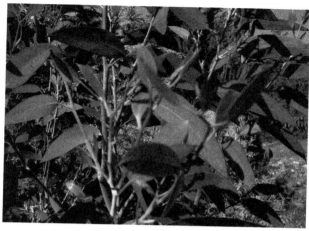

Eucalyptus oil has been applied for its healing properties and for industrial and practical uses. This pure essential oil is distilled from the dried leaves of the fast-growing evergreen tree, *Eucalyptus globulus*, that is native to Australia. At least 500 of the 700 different eucalyptus species produce a kind of essential oil.

TIP: Did you know that eucalyptus is highly effective in helping with your asthma symptoms? Simply take a paper towel and add 3-4 drops of eucalyptus oil directly on it, then lay it by your head while you sleep.

Availability: In most good herbal remedy shops. (e.g. iHerb.com, Amazon.com, naissance.co.uk)

Antibiotic Properties: Flavonoids and volatile oils, which kill bacteria. Eucalyptus is *primarily used for respiratory support (blocked nose, cough, and sinusitis)*.

Collection & Preparation: Available as an oil, essential oils, cough drops, and as a flavoring agent.

Dosage: Ensure oil products contain no more than 25% eucalyptus. External use is recommended. To treat a cough, combine a couple drops of eucalyptus oil with boiling water, then inhale the steam for 10 minutes two times daily.

Possible Side Effects: Nausea, vomiting, diarrhea, headache.

Contraindications: Do not take if pregnant, breastfeeding or you suffer from diabetes, high blood pressure, or epilepsy. Avoid applying over wounds, cuts, or broken skin. Always consult doctor before using it.

Alternatives: N/A.

Other Uses: Upset stomach, asthma, herpes, malaria, fever, bronchitis, whooping cough, gallbladder problems, cancer, oral health, etc.

28. Goldenseal

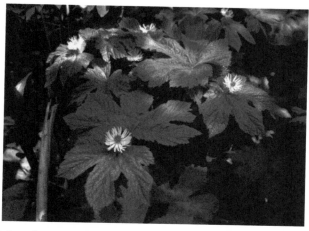

Goldenseal has been used by American Indians as an anti-inflammatory medicine to treat issues including genito-urinary tract, respiratory, or digestive inflammation (caused by either allergy or infection). Specifically, the Iroquois used a root decoction to treat pneumonia, fever, whooping cough, sour stomach, diarrhea, flatulence, and liver disease. They mixed it with whiskey to alleviate heart troubles, and added other roots to create an infusion that could work as a treatment for sore eyes and help treat earache. Whereas, the Cherokee applied this root to enhance appetite, in a decoction to alleviate general weakness, and in a wash to treat local inflammation. Therefore, goldenseal has gained the reputation of being an effective herbal antibiotic and immunity booster, helping it become one of the most popular herbs sold in America.

TIP: If you suffer from digestive tract disorders, try using goldenseal. It is a good herb to cure peptic ulcers, heartburn, diarrhea, and constipation.

Availability: In most good herbal remedy stores. (e.g. iHerb.com, Amazon.com)

Antibiotic Properties: Hydrastine, berberine, canadine, canadaline, and l-hydrastine, all of which work to kill bacteria. Goldenseal *primarily works to aid your digestive system.*

Collection & Preparation: Available as a tablet, capsule, extract, or tincture.

Dosage: 0.3-1 ml of liquid extract, 0.5-5 g capsules or tablets, or 10-20 drops of tincture – all taken 2-3 times a day. Do not take on empty stomach.

Possible Side Effects: Numbness, sickness, diarrhea, allergic reactions on skin, or throat problems.

Contraindications: Do not use if pregnant, breastfeeding or for newborn babies. Avoid using if the following health issues exist: blood pressure problems, heart problems, diabetes, glaucoma. Avoid use if allergic to ragweed. Consult a doctor before taking it.

Alternatives: N/A.

Other Uses: Food poisoning, cold and flu, eczema, cough, sinusitis, constipation, cancer, hay fever, hemorrhoids, chronic fatigue, liver problems, arrhythmia, prostatitis, etc.

29. Grapefruit Seed Extract

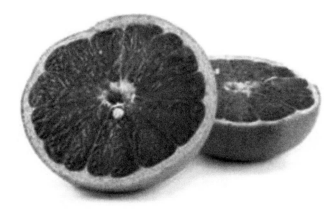

The medicinal properties of grapefruit seed extract were first documented in 1972 by physicist Dr. Jacob Harich, who noticed its use as a disinfectant in several countries. Asia, South America, and Europe have all applied the citrusy extract as an antibacterial, antiviral substance, and as a cleanser for home, hair, and skin. This sub-tropical tree grows abundantly within several countries, and the liquid extract comes from the tree's seeds and fruit.

TIP: Did you know grapefruit contains the chemical benzalkonium chloride? This helps to alleviate earache and fights ear infection. For 5-7 days, apply 1-2 drops of fresh grapefruit juice to the affected ear twice daily.

Availability: In most good health food and herbal remedy stores. (e.g. iHerb.com, Amazon.com, simplysupplements.net)

Antibiotic Properties: *Citrus racemosa*, which fights parasitic organisms and works well against a variety of bacterial infections. Grapefruit seed extract *is primarily used to harden arteries in atherosclerosis sufferers.*

Collection & Preparation: Available in a cream, juice, capsules, or tincture.

Dosage: No more than 1500 mg per day.

Possible Side Effects: Be careful with use if you're a post-menopausal woman, as in excess, it can increase your chances of getting breast cancer by 25-30%.

Contraindications: Do not use if you're suffering from breast cancer or other hormone sensitive cancers.

Alternatives: Citrus seed extract.

Other Uses: Candidiasis, yeast infections, cancer, psoriasis, bronchitis, hay fever, hair growth, fungal nails, ear problems, sore throat, gingivitis, depression, lung treatments, etc.

Grapefruit, raw, white, all areas

Nutritional value per 100 g (3.5 oz)		
Energy	138 kJ (33 kcal)	
Carbohydrates	8.41 g	
Sugars	7.31 g	
Dietary fiber	1.1 g	
Fat	0.10 g	
Protein	.8 g	
Vitamins	**Quantity**	**%DV**[†]
Thiamine (B_1)	0.037 mg	3%
Riboflavin (B_2)	0.020 mg	2%
Niacin (B_3)	0.269 mg	2%
Pantothenic acid (B_5)	0.283 mg	6%
Vitamin B_6	0.043 mg	3%
Folate (B_9)	10 µg	3%
Choline	7.7 mg	2%
Vitamin C	33.3 mg	40%
Vitamin E	0.13 mg	1%
Minerals	**Quantity**	**%DV**[†]
Calcium	12 mg	1%
Iron	0.06 mg	0%
Magnesium	9 mg	3%
Manganese	0.013 mg	1%
Phosphorus	8 mg	1%
Potassium	148 mg	3%
Zinc	0.07 mg	1%
Other constituents	**Quantity**	
Water	90.48 g	

30. Juniper

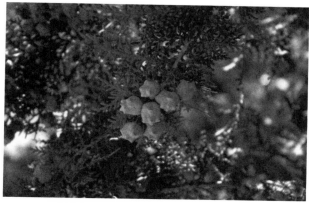

Juniper berries have disinfecting, stimulating, and warming properties that make them an effective herbal medicine. Due to their antiseptic effect, juniper berries are often applied to alleviate symptoms of chronic and recurring urinary tract infections. They can be applied between flare-ups, because juniper berries will stimulate the kidneys to quickly flush fluids. And, for those with frequent urinary infections, this can be helpful but not as effective in the acute cases. However, this same stimulation would be completely painful if you had a kidney infection. Additionally, juniper berries have been used in the treatment of prolapse and weakness of the urethra or bladder. Be aware of this herb's potential, use juniper berries carefully; begin with small amounts, and apply this herb under the thoughtful supervision of a professional herbal practitioner.

TIP: Juniper berry is a good remedy for skin problems. It removes toxins from the blood and cures acne and eczema. It can also cure other skin problems like athlete's foot and dandruff.

Availability: In most good herbal remedy stores. (e.g. iHerb.com, Amazon.com, naturessunshine.com)

Antibiotic Properties: Thujine and terpenine, which form an antiseptic barrier making them great for kidney ailments. Juniper is *primarily used for digestive disorders and it's extremely effective for enlarged prostate problems.*

Collection & Preparation: Available as an oil, tincture, or as berries that can be used in food.

Dosage: 20-100 mg of the essential oil, 2-10 g of the berries.

Possible Side Effects: Skin and respiratory allergic reactions can occur. It may also cause stomach upset.

Contraindications: Do not use if pregnant or breastfeeding. Avoid use if you suffer from diabetes, kidney diseases, stomach and intestinal disorders, or blood pressure issues.

Alternatives: N/A.

Other Uses: Heartburn, indigestion, urinary tract infections, asthma, bronchitis, joint pain, kidney and bladder stones, skin problems, etc.

31. Sage

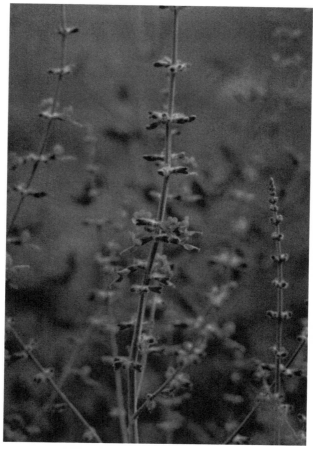

Sage has medicinal properties that can help relieve the symptoms of mental disorders, for example, depression and Alzheimer's, and digestion problems. Due to its pleasant, unique aroma, this herb has been used in cosmetics and soaps as well. Sage is a member of the Lamiaceae family along with other herbs like basil, thyme, oregano, lavender, and rosemary.

TIP: Did you know that sage slows down the brain aging and speeds up the transmission of brain signals? Brew a tea from the leaves or chew on 2-3 leaves once daily to boost memory.

Availability: In most good herbal remedy stores. (e.g. healthspan.co.uk, iHerb.com, Amazon.com)

Antibiotic Properties: Escherichia coli, salmonella typhi, s. enteritidis, and shigella sonnei, which have the power to constrict, so it is *primarily used for* *stomach issues and candidiasis.*

Collection & Preparation: Available as a capsule, cream, or an herb for food. Can be made into a tea by placing a teaspoon of powdered or fresh sage in boiling water. Can be made into a tonic by pouring a quart of boiling water over a handful of leaves and leave it to stew overnight.

Dosage: 1-2.5 g three times a day.

Possible Side Effects: Restlessness, irritability, headaches, stomach upset, dizziness, epilepsy.

Contraindications: Do not use if you suffer from diabetes, epilepsy, high blood pressure, or seizure disorders, also if pregnant or breastfeeding.

Alternatives: Rosemary.

Other Uses: Sore throat, stomach pain, difficult menses, cold, menopause side effects, bloating, memory loss, overproduction of saliva, Alzheimer's, etc.

32. Wormwood

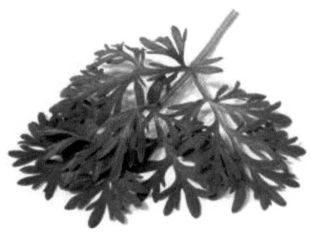

Wormwood's most common use is to aid in digestion with its bitter taste, which provokes the gallbladder to release bile, among other secretions from other intestinal glands. This process enables the body to digest food, so people who don't produce enough stomach acid, or experience weak digestion, would directly benefit from this herb. It's digestion-boosting properties are so strong, it can cause diarrhea and has been used to help the body expel parasites such as pinworms and roundworms. Be aware that his herb should only be used in small dosages over a short time because wormwood contains a substance that becomes toxic when consumed over a long period of time.

TIP: Wormwood is a great remedy to expel Ascaris. Make a powder of wormwood, and take 1 tablespoon two times a day.

Availability: Most good herbal remedy stores. (e.g. iHerb.com, Amazon.com)

Antibiotic Properties: Thujone and isothujone, which work to stimulate the gallbladder making it extremely beneficial to the digestive system. Wormwood is *primarily used for stomach upset and digestive disorders.*

Collection & Preparation: Available as a powder for tea, a capsule, a tablet, tincture, or an essential oil.

Dosage: Tea = 1 teaspoon of powder mixed with boiling water, steep for 15 minutes, then drink before eating. Capsule = one before meal times (three times a day). Tincture = 1/8 of a teaspoon before meals. Do not take in large doses.

Possible Side Effects: Thirst, numbness, sickness, restlessness, nightmares, nausea, diarrhea, and kidney issues. Prolonged use may prove toxic.

Contraindications: Do not use if you suffer from allergy to ragweed, kidney disorders, seizure disorders, porphyria or are pregnant or breastfeeding.

Alternatives: N/A.

Other Uses: Gallbladder problems, insect bites, liver disease, worm infections, anemia, Candida albicans, etc.

33. Thyme

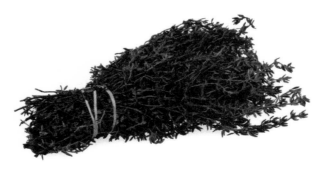

Thyme's leaves, flowers, and the extracted oil can be used as a diuretic and for treating flatulence, bronchitis, bedwetting, stomachache, diarrhea, colic, cough and pertussis, sore throat, and arthritis. This herb also has culinary and ornamental uses.

TIP: Did you know that thyme stimulates and tones up the nervous system, such as neurasthenia, depression, nightmares, nervous exhaustion, insomnia, and melancholy?

Availability: Most good health food and herbal remedy stores. (e.g. iHerb.com, Amazon.com)

Antibiotic Properties: Thymol, which works to suppress inflammatory cyclooxygenase-2. This means thyme is *primarily used for coughs, colds, and feverish symptoms.*

Collection & Preparation: Can be used in food, or available as an oil or tincture. Can be made into a tea by mixing the leaves with boiling water, which can make a great replacement for coffee for a healthier lifestyle. Extracted oil, however, should not be taken internally because it is considered highly toxic.

Dosage: For cough – syrup of thyme can be taken orally for five days, for upper respiratory tract infections – a tea made by 1-2 g dried herb steeped in 150 ml boiling water for 10 minutes, then drink several times per day. Other uses – 20-40 drops of liquid extract three times daily in juice; 40 drops of tincture up to three times daily.

Possible Side Effects: Digestive system upset, headache, dizziness.

Contraindications: Do not take if you suffer from oregano allergies; suffer from bleeding disorders, heart problems, epilepsy, high blood pressure, and hormone sensitive disorders. Avoid during pregnancy and breastfeeding.

Alternatives: Oregano.

Other Uses: Acne, colic, anemia, asthma, gastrointestinal disorders, yeast infection, cancer, snakebites, skin issues, neuralgia, etc.

34. Green Tea

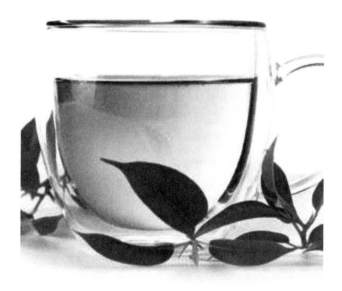

Green tea leaves are believed to have a higher concentration of antioxidants, due to the way they are processed. These leaves contain antioxidants such as caffeine, B vitamins, manganese, folate (natural version of folic acid), potassium, magnesium, and catechins. It is this health property that has driven green tea's use for centuries, especially within traditional Chinese medicine, as a treatment for everything from depression to headaches. Green tea has also been used to prevent Alzheimer's disease and cancer, enhance weight loss, fight cardiovascular disease, and reduce cholesterol. Black, green, and oolong teas originate from the *Camellia sinensis* plant. Steamed fresh leaves produce green tea, while fermentation of the leaves produce oolong and black teas.

TIP: Did you know that green tea is much better than coffee? Here's why:

- Includes more antioxidant and anticancer compounds.

- Fights obesity by boosting metabolism and being low-calorie.

- Hydrates your body more quickly.

- Provides longer-lasting energy.

- Is ideal stress treatment by relaxing your brain and calming your nerves.

- Reduces osteoporosis risk by supporting bone formation.

- Boosts your immunity against germs, viruses, and infections.

Availability: In most good health food and herbal remedy stores.

Antibiotic Properties: *Camellia sinensis*, which actually works well alongside conventional antibiotics to fight off bugs. Green tea is *primarily used for high blood pressure and digestive disorders.*

Collection & Preparation: Available as tea leaves or tea bags. Brew the tea by mixing 2 oz of leaves with 6 oz of water. Green tea is also available as a capsule or tablet to be taken 3-4 times daily.

Dosage: No more than 3 cups a day.

Possible Side Effects: Headaches, nervousness, sleep problems, constipation, dizziness, and irritability.

Contraindications: Avoid using when pregnant or breastfeeding or if you suffer from blood pressure issues. Do not consume more than 2 cups daily if you have an irregular heart beat or anxiety disorder.

Alternatives: N/A.

Other Uses: Cataract, dental diseases, rosacea, cancer, obesity and weight loss, baldness, cholesterol, Alzheimer's, etc.

35. Ashwagandha (Withania Somnifera)

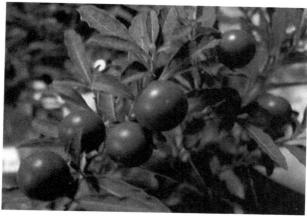

Ashwagandha has been in use since the ancient times, being known for its restorative properties and in treating various conditions. It is still considered one of the most powerful herbs used in Ayurvedic healing. Traditionally, it has been applied to boost immune systems post-illness. Ashwagandha translates to "the smell of a horse"; in common use, that means the herb can bestow the strength and vigor of a stallion.

Ashwagandha is a plump shrub with yellow flowers and oval leaves, which belongs to the Solanaceae family. Its fruit is red and grows to about the same size as a raisin. Native to the drier regions of the Middle East, northern Africa, and India, today, it is also growing in more mild climates, such as North America.

TIP: Are you facing problems with poor memory; are you stressed from your day to day work? The solution is ashwagandha. It relaxes the body, minimizes chronic stress, and enhances learning power by enhancing the memory. It will also enhance stamina, strength, and energy of the body.

Availability: In most good herbal remedy stores. (e.g. iHerb.com, Amazon.com)

Antibiotic Properties: Glycoprotein, which helps calm the brain, reduce swelling, and boost the immune system. Ashwagandha is *primarily used for stress relief and hypothyroidism.*

Collection & Preparation: Typically, ashwagandha is consumed in powder form, but it can also be taken as capsules. Boil 1 level teaspoon of the powder in 1 cup of milk over low heat for 10 minutes. Add 1 teaspoon of a natural sweetener, such as honey, and 1/4 teaspoon of spice, such as ginger or cinnamon. Enhance ashwagandha's effect by including 1/2 teaspoon of ghee (or clarified butter).

Dosage: Initially begin with smaller dose to see if it suits your body. Take 2 g twice a day from 1-3 months. It is advised to take a break of one or two weeks after consuming it for two straight months. For leaves in powder form, take 3-5 g; for root in powder form, take 1/4 to 1/2 of a tablespoon.

Possible Side Effects: Stomach upset, diarrhea and vomiting, drowsiness, low blood pressure, lower blood sugar, abdominal pain, shallow breathing.

Contraindications: Do not use if you suffer from diabetes, congestion, blood pressure issues, stomach ulcers, or autoimmune diseases. Avoid during pregnancy or breastfeeding. Do not take ashwagandha if you're allergic to it (if you're unable to digest tomatoes, potatoes, or peppers, you should avoid this herb). Ashwagandha may adversely affect the actions of some medications, hence you should consult your doctor before taking it.

Alternatives: Shatavari.

Other Uses: Alzheimer's, anxiety, fatigue, lack of concentration, stabilizes blood sugar, lower cholesterol, anemia, cancer, anorexia, arthritis, etc.

36. Atractylodes

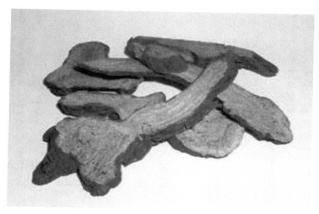

Atractylodes is an herb taken from Chinese tonic herbalism, and it is important there for its work in building Qi – a circulating life force important to Chinese medicine and philosophy. This herb is used as an energy tonic and for regulating digestion. Even though it is neither rare or expensive, atractylodes is highly regarded for its medicinal benefits.

Availability: In most good herbal remedy stores. (e.g. Amazon.com)

Antibiotic Properties: *Cang zhu*, which works alongside your immune system, making it great for stomach upset. Atractylodes is *primarily used for indigestion and other digestive disorders.*

Collection & Preparation: Available in medicinal form (powder, tincture, or essential oil).

Dosage: 10-30 drops of tincture, 2-3 times a day. It is considered safe when not exceeding 1.32 g daily and being taken up to seven weeks.

Possible Side Effects: Nausea, dry mouth, and bad taste in your mouth.

Contraindications: Avoid using if you have an allergy to ragweed or you have yin deficiency with heat signs and extreme thirst. Avoid use during pregnancy and breastfeeding.

Alternatives: A. chinensis, A. japonicum, and A. ovate.

Other Uses: Repeated miscarriage, weight loss due to cancer, bloating, cancer, joint pain, etc.

37. Ginseng

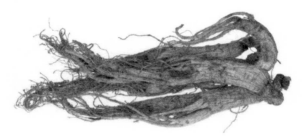

Ginseng has been applied in the treatment of several medical conditions, but only a few treatments can be supported by validated research. However, studies have shown that among the varieties of ginseng, each type provides its own benefit. Among those varieties, two strains of ginseng are the most popular: American (*Panax quinquefolius*) and Korean or Asian (*Panax ginseng*). In traditional Chinese medicine, Korean ginseng is considered the stronger strain, more than the American strain. Be aware that other herbs get called "ginseng" – such as Siberian ginseng or eleuthero – but they lack the active ginsenosides ingredient.

TIP: Did you know that ginseng helps to avoid early aging? The herb has a mental stimulant effect in aged people and bolsters the memory and cognitive power of the elderly. It also energizes the body and alleviates tiredness.

Availability: In most good herbal remedy stores. (e.g. iHerb.com, Amazon.com, simplysupplements.net)

Antibiotic Properties: Ginsenosides, which work on many of the areas of the body and helps improve the body's resistance to stress and increases vitality. Ginseng is *primarily used to fight respiratory tract infections, debility, and diabetes.*

Collection & Preparation: Available as a capsule, powder, tincture, tablet or can be taken as a tea from fresh root or dried root powder.

Dosage: Dry root – 1 g daily, and don't take for longer than three months at a time. Then a break of one week to three months is recommended.

Possible Side Effects: Nervousness, insomnia, anxiety, hypertension, rise in blood sugar, edema, headaches, and stomach upset.

Contraindications: Do not take if you suffer from diabetes, autoimmune diseases; are on Warfarin or antidepressants, or experience an acute fever or sore throat. Avoid while pregnant or breastfeeding. Not recommended for children or if you plan surgery within ten days or less. Always discuss with health practitioner before using it.

Alternatives: Rhodiola.

Other Uses: Stress, fatigue, to increase energy levels, anemia, anti-aging, diabetes, cold, Alzheimer's, heart diseases, high cholesterol, cancer, fibromyalgia, etc.

38. Greater Celandine

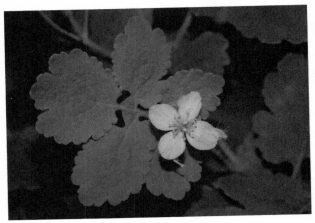

Greater celandine, or *Chelidonium majus*, has a long, recorded history of medicinal use throughout many European countries. Dioscorides, Pliny the Elder, and ancient Greeks, in general, considered celandine an effective detoxifying agent. Additionally, the Romans applied celandine to cleanse blood, and Maurice Mességué, a French herbalist, recommended celandine tea to provide relief for liver problems. Celandine has also been used within traditional Chinese medicine, and it has become an important element within Western phytotherapy. Greater celandine extracts have exhibited liver-protecting potential alongside toxicity on a broad spectrum toward harmful organisms. This has generated the inclusion of greater celandine within gallbladder and liver cleansing and support regimens.

TIP: This herb is very effective in treating warts. Treat two or three warts by applying fresh juice 2-3 times daily dabbed on a cotton ball. Take note, this juice is toxic; it can blister the skin. So, dab no more than two or three warts during each application.

Availability: In most good herbal remedy stores. (e.g. iHerb.com, Amazon.com)

Antibiotic Properties: Alkaloids and flavonoids, which encourage a stronger immune system and aids digestion. Greater celandine is *primarily used for digestive tract issues*.

Collection & Preparation: Available as a cream or a tincture. The roots are used to create this medicine.

Dosage: The cream can be applied as needed. The tincture, 10-20 drops twice a day for four weeks.

Possible Side Effects: The cream can cause a skin rash. High dosage can cause breathing problems, sleepiness, and coughing.

Contraindications: Do not use if you suffer from autoimmune diseases, diarrhea, liver disease, hepatitis or if you have a bile duct blockage. Avoid giving to children; also avoid if pregnant or breastfeeding.

Alternatives: N/A.

Other Uses: Jaundice, high blood pressure, hepatitis, cancer, anxiety, arthritis, warts, IBS, constipation, menstrual cramps, pain, etc.

39. Shatavari

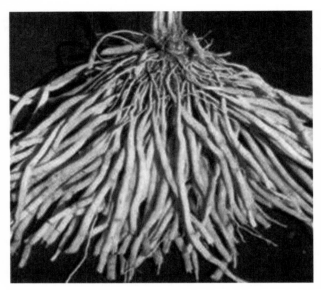

Shatavari offers healing properties to treat a variety of ailments that affect both men and women. Also known as *Asparagus racemosus*, shatavari is a climbing plant that grows throughout India in low jungle regions. It is a sweet and bitter herb, which Indians think of as the women's equivalent to ashwagandha. The name 'Shatavari' translates to "she who possesses 100 husbands," which refers to the herb's rejuvenation effect on the female reproductive organs.

TIP: Did you know that shatavari reduces the regular complaints of women? It is helpful to women in all aspects: tones the system and supports women at the beginning of menses, during ovulation, by strengthening the uterus during pregnancy and birth, and by inducing lactation.

Availability: In most good herbal remedy stores. (e.g. iHerb.com, Amazon.com, pukkaherbs.com)

Antibiotic Properties: Saponins, which increase antibacterial activity in the body making it great for fighting off and preventing bacterial infections. Shatavari is *primarily used for digestive tract issues or hysterectomy and oophorectomy*.

Collection & Preparation: Available as a powder, juice or in tablet or capsule form.

Dosage: 1/2 to 1 teaspoon of the powder mixed with milk twice daily. Tablets and capsules to be taken 2-3 times daily.

Possible Side Effects: Dizziness, fatigue, and weight gain.

Contraindications: Do not use if you suffer from kidney disorders or lung congestion. Always consult a doctor before using it.

Alternatives: Ashwagandha.

Other Uses: Fluid retention, menstrual disorders, dysentery, stress, diarrhea, rheumatism, headaches, coughs, alcohol withdrawal, etc.

40. Shiitake

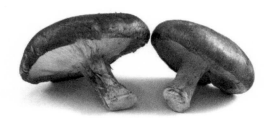

Shiitake mushrooms have long been considered a symbol of longevity in Asia due to their inherent medicinal properties. This health-supporting fungus, lacking roots, seeds, leaves, or flowers, has been applied by the Chinese in healing treatments for at least 6,000 years. But it has been their rich, smoky flavor that has put them on supermarket shelves across the U.S.

Availability: In most good health food and herbal remedy stores. (e.g. iHerb.com, Amazon.com, swansonvitamins.com)

Antibiotic Properties: *Lentinula edodes*, which kills off a wide range of bacterial pathogens. Shiitake is *primarily used to work against immune system failure.*

Collection & Preparation: Can be consumed with food or taken as an extract or capsules and powder.

Dosage: Extract = 1-3 g taken three times a day. 6-16 g of the whole, dried shiitake mushroom can be ingested daily. Capsules can be taken three times daily for six months and 4 g of shiitake powder for ten weeks.

Possible Side Effects: Stomach discomfort, diarrhea, inflammation, skin reactions, breathing problems. It may cause bladder cancer.

Contraindications: Do not use if you suffer from autoimmune diseases or eosinophilia. Avoid if pregnant or breastfeeding.

Alternatives: Maitake.

Other Uses: Cholesterol levels, tumors, cancer, bronchitis, angina, asthma, flu, anti-aging, etc.

Mushrooms, shiitake, dried

Nutritional value per 100 g (3.5 oz)

Energy	1,238 kJ (296 kcal)
Carbohydrates	75.37 g
Sugars	2.21 g
Dietary fiber	11.5 g
Fat	0.99 g
Protein	9.58 g

Vitamins	Quantity	%DV[†]
Thiamine (B$_1$)	0.3 mg	26%
Riboflavin (B$_2$)	1.27 mg	106%
Niacin (B$_3$)	14.1 mg	94%
Pantothenic acid (B$_5$)	21.879 mg	438%
Vitamin B$_6$	0.965 mg	74%
Folate (B$_9$)	163 µg	41%
Vitamin C	3.5 mg	4%
Vitamin D	3.9 µg	26%

Minerals	Quantity	%DV[†]
Calcium	11 mg	1%
Iron	1.72 mg	13%
Magnesium	132 mg	37%
Manganese	1.176 mg	56%
Phosphorus	294 mg	42%
Potassium	1534 mg	33%
Sodium	13 mg	1%
Zinc	7.66 mg	81%

Other constituents	Quantity
Water	9.5 g
Selenium	46 ug

41. Ginkgo Biloba

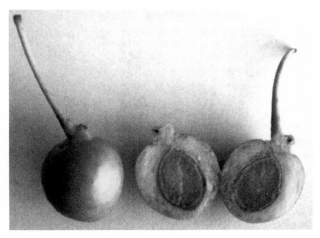

Ginkgo biloba is an ancient herb with properties that enhance oxygen utilization, concentration, memory, along with other mental facilities and provides medicinal benefits, especially alleviating depression symptoms, for the elderly. Additionally, ginkgo has the potential for reversing retina damage, boosting long-distance vision, and relieving symptoms of vertigo, sinusitis, tinnitus, and headache. The history of ginkgo biloba use has been traced back almost 300 million years, which makes it the oldest tree species still growing on earth. Commonly called the maidenhair tree, the plant has been used in China across hundreds of years for medicinal purposes, however, the modern applications are based on German research, where ginkgo is a prescription herb.

TIP: Did you know that this herb helps with deep vein thrombosis? Ginkgo dilates the blood vessels and helps to improve the blood flow. The flavonoids present in gingko reduce the numbness and swelling in the legs due to the deep vein thrombosis. Take gingko capsules of 60 mg twice a day for a month.

Availability: In most good herbal remedy stores. (e.g. iHerb.com, Amazon.com, woodshealth.com)

Antibiotic Properties: Ginkgolides, bilobalides, and flavonoids, which improve blood circulation and kill bacteria. Ginkgo biloba is *primarily used for diseases that slow the body down.*

Collection & Preparation: Available in capsule, tincture, and tablet forms.

Dosage: 120-240 mg per day. The dosage depends on the illness you are trying to combat. It is recommended to reduce the dose after ten days.

Possible Side Effects: Stomach upset, headache, dizziness, drowsiness, constipation, forceful heartbeat, high or low blood pressure, and allergic skin reactions.

Contraindications: Do not use if you suffer from diabetes, seizures, infertility, bleeding disorders or for children. Avoid if pregnant or breastfeeding.

Alternatives: N/A.

Other Uses: Atherosclerosis, dizziness, tinnitus, impotence, dementia, Lyme disease, vertigo, mood disturbances, Alzheimer's, asthma, Raynaud's syndrome, etc.

42. Neem (Margosa)

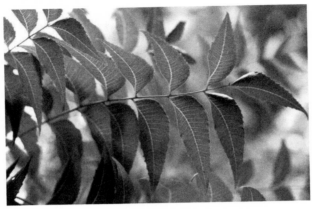

Everyday use of neem is on the rise, as more research is conducted to validate the medicinal properties of this tree and its extracts. Native to Asia, this ancient tree has been a natural source of medicinal compounds across thousands of years – as far back as the beginning of Hinduism. Indian farmers have purposefully harvested this valuable herbal aid for its beneficial uses from far back as the Vedic period, 1500-600 B.C. Into the modern era, neem has been applied externally and internally with traditional Ayurvedic herbal treatments throughout India. This herbal product has expanded out to other parts of the world; American and European scientists have studied the potential medical benefits of neem. As more studies return positive results, more people will learn about neem and how it supports daily living, regular health regimens and alleviates general irritation and ailments.

TIP: Did you know that neem has been used since ancient times to treat many skin problems. It has a soothing effect on irritating skin and acts as a nutritive tonic to the skin by treating eczema, dandruff, rashes, and ringworm. It is used as a face pack to cure pimples, redness, and scars. Treating skin diseases, start with 250 g of mustard oil and boil it in an iron pan. Mix in 50 g of soft neem leaves; cook until the leaves have turned black; cool and strain the oil. Apply directly to the affected area three times daily.

Availability: In most good herbal remedy stores. (e.g. theneemteam.co.uk, iHerb.com, Amazon.com)

Antibiotic Properties: Sulfurous compounds, polyphenolics such as flavonoids and their glycosides, dihydrochalcone, coumarin and tannins, aliphatic compounds, which work to boost your body's immune system making them great for liver problems. Neem is *primarily used for cardiovascular diseases and skin problems.*

Collection & Preparation: Available as an oil, extract, tincture, capsules, and tea made by mixing the leaves with boiling water.

Dosage: Capsules = 1-2 twice a day; and oil/tincture = 5 drops daily.

Possible Side Effects: If taken for a long period of time, it can harm your kidneys and liver. Can cause stomach irritation.

Contraindications: Do not use if you are trying to conceive, or suffer from autoimmune disorders, diabetes, or have had an organ transplant. Avoid if pregnant or breastfeeding.

Alternatives: N/A.

Other Uses: Leprosy, hepatitis B, candidiasis, body lice, blackheads, dandruff, eye disorders, gum disease, hemorrhoids, blood vessels, etc.

43. Propolis

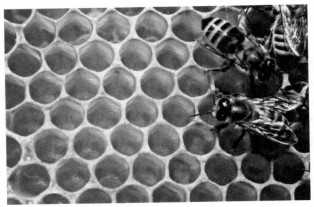

Propolis and its medicinal properties have a long history stemming from its use by ancient civilizations. Egyptians used it while embalming mummies; Assyrians used it to fight infection and heal wounds, tumors; the Greeks used it in the treatment of abscesses. This herbal compound is produced by bees and their use of the sap from evergreens or needle-leaved trees. A sticky, green-brown product is generated, which is usually applied to coat the hives, as the bees combine their beeswax and other natural discharges with the sap.

The bees' location and the selection of flowers and trees will have a direct effect on the propolis's composition. For instance, propolis harvested in China isn't going to have the same chemical composition as that harvested in New Zealand. Determining the compound's health benefits with any certainty is made more complex due to those inherent differences.

TIP: You can use propolis-rich lip balm on your lips to treat oral herpes.

Availability: In most herbal remedy stores. (e.g. iHerb.com, Amazon.com)

Antibiotic Properties: Galangin, which creates a sterile environment that helps boost your immune system. Propolis is *primarily used for infections caused by bacteria, e.g. TB (Tuberculosis)*.

Collection & Preparation: Available as a cream, oil, and capsules.

Dosage: Cream = 3% ointment; capsule = 500 mg per day.

Possible Side Effects: Irritation.

Contraindications: Avoid using when you're pregnant or breastfeeding, or if you suffer from asthma, bleeding conditions, or honey allergies.

Alternatives: Honey-based products.

Other Uses: Coryza, canker sores, nose and throat cancer, peptic ulcer disease, ear discharge, herpes, cold sores, etc.

44. Sanguinaria (Bloodroot)

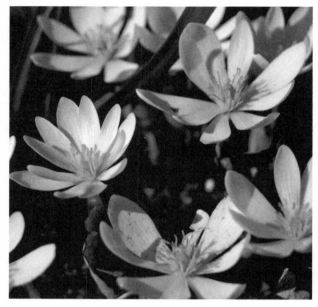

Sanguinaria has been applied medicinally for its antioxidant, anti-inflammatory, and antimicrobial properties. Specifically, it is an additive in toothpastes and antiseptic mouth rinses to alleviate gingival inflammation and dental plaque. Additionally, this plant alkaloid has been found to hinder platelet aggregation caused by collagen, arachidonic acid, and a sub-threshold thrombin concentration. Sanguinaria is found in the root of *Sanguinaria canadensis* and the *Poppy fumaria* species. It is defined as a cationic molecule that can convert to an alkanolamine form at pH greater than 7 from an iminium ion form at pH less than 6. Along with other alkaloids, sanguinaria comprises the active ingredients in most sanguinaria extracts.

TIP: Blood root is a great herbal treatment for skin conditions like warts and moles. When you apply sanguinaria directly to the wounds, it removes the damaged tissues.

Availability: In most good herbal remedy stores. (e.g. iHerb.com, Amazon.com)

Antibiotic Properties: Sanguinarine alkaloids, chelerythrine, protopine, and B. homochelidonine, which actually inhibits the bacteria before killing it. Sanguinaria is *primarily used for oral problems*.

Collection & Preparation: Available as a tincture, a powder, toothpaste, and a fluid.

Dosage: Tincture = 10-15 drops; powder = 1 grain; and fluid = 10-30 drops daily.

Possible Side Effects: Nausea, vomiting, drowsiness, vertigo, burning in the stomach, low blood pressure.

Contraindications: Do not use if you suffer from intestinal problems or glaucoma. Avoid if pregnant or breastfeeding.

Alternatives: N/A.

Other Uses: Croup, bronchitis, skin problems, warts, nasal polyps, achy joints, gum disease, poor circulation, high blood pressure, headache, cancer, etc.

45. Tea Tree

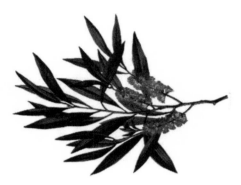

Tea tree oil has medicinal benefits that have recently been confirmed by the scientific community, but it has been in use for thousands of years by aborigine tribes as a general antiseptic and as a natural antibacterial disinfectant. These properties make it effective in fighting viruses, bacteria, and fungus, and it's capable of fighting several infections that are otherwise resistant to antibiotics. So it has become a natural remedy for minor wounds, irritations, and bacterial and fungal ailments, including athlete's foot, abscess, acne, warts, dandruff, herpes, rashes, insect bites, blisters, oily skin, and sun burns. Also known as melaleuca, tea tree oil is light yellow in color with a scent reminiscent of nutmeg. The oil is extracted by steaming the leaves, then squeezing out the oil.

TIP: Tea tree oil is great for curing warts. Soak a cotton ball in tea tree oil and apply it carefully to the affected area. Repeat daily for 8-10 days.

Availability: Most good herbal remedy stores. (e.g. hollandandbarrett.com, iHerb.com, Amazon.com)

Antibiotic Properties: *Melaleuca alternifolia*, which 'punches holes' in bacteria to kill them. Tea tree oil is *primarily used for skin issues*.

Collection & Preparation: Available as an essential oil. This oil can be made by distilling the leaves.

Dosage: The percent of the oil depends on your issue – please consult with your doctor. Always dilute tea tree oil in some carrier oil in the ratio of 1:10.

Possible Side Effects: Itchiness, irritation, redness, drowsiness, stomach upset.

Contraindications: Do not use if you're pregnant or breastfeeding. Avoid using around eyes, swallowing, or absorbing it.

Alternatives: N/A.

Other Uses: Inflamed gums, abscess, laryngitis, cough, cold, candidiasis, acrochordon, dandruff, plaque, etc.

Tea tree oil composition, as per ISO 4730 (2017)[1]

Component	Concentration
terpinen-4-ol	35.0–48.0%
γ-terpinene	14–28%
α-terpinene	6.0–12.0%
1,8-cineole	traces–10.0%
terpinolene	1.5–5.0%
α-terpineol	2.0–5.0%
α-pinene	1.0–4.0%
p-Cymene	0.5–8.0%
Sabinene	traces–3.5%
limonene	0.5–1.5%
aromadendrene	0.2–3.0%
ledene	0.1–3.0%
globulol	traces–1.0%
viridiflorol	traces–1.0%

Of course, there are many amazing herbs with antibiotic uses and other health benefits. This list is just the start of the things that can help you! Further research can assist you if it is an area that interests you. There are many online resources with information, some of which are listed later in this guide.

Tip: iHerb.com has most of the herbal antibiotics you might be looking for, at very affordable prices. Make sure to take advantage of $5 off for the first order with the following voucher code: **WCR736**.

CHAPTER 7

LITTLE KNOWN HERBAL REMEDY RECIPES

This chapter is going to look at a few **herbal remedy recipes for common ailments** that you can create at home.

1. Vitamin C Pills

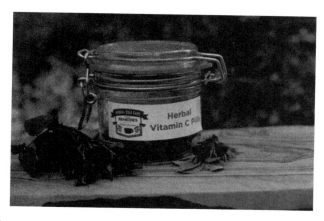

Used for:

Vitamin C tablets are useful for helping to boost the immune system and fight off colds and flu-like symptoms.

Ingredients:

- 1 tablespoon of rose hip powder (*the fruit of a rose plant, which has a high Vitamin C content*)

- 1 tablespoon of amla powder (*an Indian gooseberry, which has strong antibacterial properties*)

- 1 tablespoon of acerola powder (*a Barbados cherry, which is great for stomach discomfort*)

- Honey

- Orange peel powder (optional) (*orange is a citrus fruit and its peel is often used for flavor*)

Instructions:

Blend the powdered herbs, smoothing out any clumped powder. Pour a few droplets of slightly warmed honey into the powdered mix. Stir, add a few more droplets, and stir again. Mix until the combination holds together, without being too sticky or moist.

Shape the mix into pea-size balls. Roll these around in the orange powder if you've selected to use it. The mixture should make 45 balls. Store these in an air-tight container to give them an extended shelf life. Take 1-3 daily.

2. Hyssop Oxymel

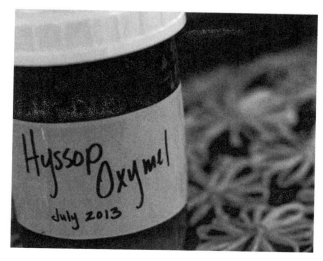

Used for:

Great for colds, flu, and bronchitis.

Ingredients:

– Hyssop (fresh or dried) (*an herbaceous plant with antiseptic and expectorant properties*)

– Honey

– Apple Cider Vinegar (*vinegar made from cider that is great for weight loss and heart health*)

Instructions:

Fill a jar lightly with chopped fresh hyssop. (Only half fill it if you're using dried hyssop). Then, fill the jar with honey just 1/3 of the way, and top it off with the apple cider vinegar. Let it sit for 2-4 weeks in the sealed jar before straining.

For a congested cough, you can take 1-2 teaspoons of this remedy every hour. Keep the hyssop oxymel in the fridge for better preservation.

3. Oatstraw Infusion

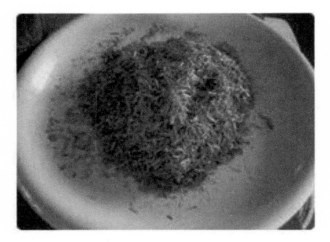

Used For:

This oatstraw infusion is great for its calming, stress relieving effect.

Ingredients:

- 1 oz of the oatstraw herb (*comes from Avena sativa, which has long-lasting energy effects*)
- Boiling water

Instructions:

Put oatstraw into a 1-quart jar, then pour boiling water over the herb. Cap it with an air-tight lid. Allow the mix to rest for 4-6 hours, which will infuse the minerals throughout the solution. Strain it. If you choose to, you can add a little extra to your mixture once it's made; lavender, lemon verbena, rosemary, etc.

Oatstraw can be used as a base for juices, lemonades, and frozen concentrates. You can use it to create ice cubes or ice pops if you want a variation.

4. Lemon Balm Home Remedy

Used For:

Perfect for cold sore sufferers as a natural way to help prevent and get rid of the virus's effects.

Ingredients:

- 2 teaspoons dried lemon balm (alternate: 2 lemon balm tea bags)
- 1 cup water, boiled

Instructions:

Boil water, then steep lemon balm for 10-15 minutes. Strain. Use a soaked cotton ball to apply mixture directly on the cold sore. Use at least 4 times daily. Alternately, try consuming a couple cups of the tea per day to help expel the virus.

5. Meadowsweet Elixir

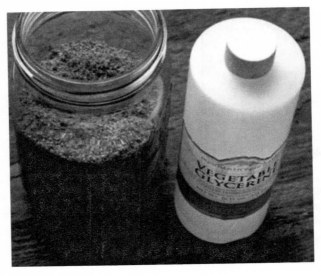

Used For:

This is a fantastic home remedy for pain relief.

Ingredients:

- 100 g of meadowsweet flowers (*a European flower that is known as 'the stomach corrector'*)
- 40 ml of 50% vodka (*a distilled alcoholic drink that consists primarily of water and ethanol*)
- 100 ml glycerin (*a sugar-alcohol compound often used in elixirs and skin care products*)

Instructions:

Place the meadowsweet flowers in a jar, and then add the vodka and glycerin. Shake well and let it macerate for 4-6 weeks. Check the mixture often, as sometimes the flowers will soak up the alcohol and glycerin so that the liquid no longer covers the herb. In this case, you either need to use a stone to weigh them down, or add more alcohol. After the 4-6 weeks, you need to strain the mixture to be ready for use.

6. Elderberry Gummy Bears

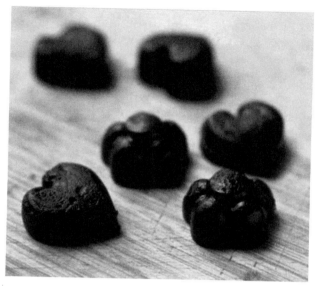

Used For:

These Vitamin C treats are good for an immune system-boosting treat that looks after your well-being.

Ingredients:

- 50 g of dried elderberries
- 30 g of dried rosehips
- 15 g of cinnamon chips
- 7 g of licorice root
- 0.5 g of freshly ground pepper (*a flowering vine, which is often used for seasoning*)
- 3 cups of apple cider
- 3 tablespoons of gelatin (*derived from collagen and used as a gelling agent in food*)

Instructions:

Place all of the ingredients (minus the gelatin) into a medium-size saucepan. Bring the mixture to simmer and continue to simmer for 20 minutes. Strain – squeeze well to extract the juice.

Measure 2 cups of juice (you can add more apple cider to make the mixture fill 2 cups). Put 1/2 cup into the fridge, then after it's chilled, dust the gelatin on top of it. Allow this to sit for one minute.

Bring the rest of the mixture to a simmer. Combine the hot juice with the cooled gelatin mixture. Stir quickly with a whisk. Continue to mix until the gelatin is completely dissolved. If you want to sweeten this up more, add sugar or honey.

Pour this mixture into molds and refrigerate. Once they have hardened, they are ready to eat. Eat 1-3 gummies per day, and keep them stored in a sealed container in the fridge.

7. Bitter Digestive Pastilles

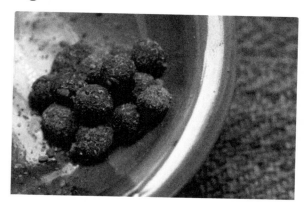

Used For:

For sufferers of bitter deficiency syndrome or for promoting a healthy digestive system.

Ingredients:

- 1/2 teaspoon of angelica root powder (*a European herb used for gastrointestinal tract disorders*)
- 1/4 teaspoon of gentian root powder (*grows in Alpine habitats and treats digestive issues*)
- 1/4 teaspoon of coriander powder (*great for promoting healthy digestion*)
- 1/4 teaspoon of orange peel powder
- 1/8 teaspoon of black pepper, freshly ground
- 1 teaspoon of natural sweetener (for example, honey)
- 1 teaspoon of powdered fennel seed (*contains anethole and polymers, which help stomach issues*)
- 1/8 teaspoon of fine sea salt (*primarily used for flavor*)

Instructions:

Mix all of the powdered herbs – except the fennel seed powder and the sea salt – in a bowl. Then, gently heat up the honey in a small saucepan just until it is thinner and more syrupy. Little by little, pour the honey into the powdered herbal mixture, constantly stirring until it can be molded into pea-shaped balls.

Roll these balls into the fennel seed powder and sea salt to create a coating. Store these in an airtight container and enjoy one 15 minutes before each meal.

8. Echinacea Remedy

Used For:

This remedy is perfect for canker sores.

Ingredients:

- 2 tablespoons tincture of sage
- 2 tablespoons tincture of echinacea
- 2 tablespoons tincture of lemon balm

Instructions:

Combine the three tinctures in a dropper bottle. Use one dropper full of the mixture to swish around your mouth 2-3 times daily.

9. Homemade Mouthwash

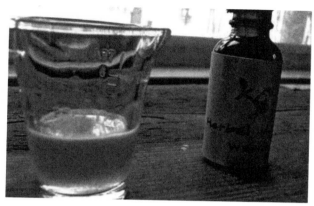

Used For:

This mixture is a great way to keep your mouth fresh and healthy.

Ingredients:

- 1/2 ounce tincture of echinacea
- 1/4 ounce tincture of Oregon grape root
- 1/8 ounce tincture of plantain (*generally used for cooking due to its sweet taste*)
- 1/8 ounce tincture of propolis

Instructions:

Mix all of the tinctures together in a bottle. Add 30-60 drops to 1 mouthful of water. Swish it in your mouth for 20-30 seconds.

10. Chamomile Remedy

Used For:

The remedy is brilliant for clearing a stuffy nose. Repeat as needed.

Ingredients:

- 2 handfuls of dried chamomile flowers/10 chamomile teabags (*a relaxing, rejuvenating herb*)
- Boiled water

Instructions:

Boil 2 quarts of water, then turn off the heat and put in the dried chamomile flowers. Cover the pot and leave for 15 minutes before placing it on a heat pad. Place a towel over your head as you breathe in the steam by leaning over the pot; this will help unblock your sinuses.

CHAPTER 8
HERBAL REMEDIES FOR COMMON AILMENTS

Ailment	Herb
Acne	Calendula, aloe, tea tree
Alcoholism	Evening primrose, kudzu
Allergy	Chamomile
Alzheimer's disease	Ginkgo, rosemary
Angina	Hawthorn, garlic, willow, green tea
Anxiety and stress	Hops, kava, passionflower, valerian, chamomile, lavender
Arteriosclerosis	Garlic
Arthritis	Capsicum, ginger, turmeric, willow, cat's claw, devil's claw
Asthma	Coffee, ephedra, tea
Athlete's foot	Topical tea tree oil
Attention-deficit disorder	Evening primrose oil

Bad breath	Parsley
Boils	Tea tree oil, topical garlic, echinacea, eleutherococcus, ginseng, rhodiola
Bronchitis	Echinacea, pelargonium
Burns	Aloe
Cancer	Bilberry, blackberry, cocoa (dark chocolate), green tea, garlic, ginseng, maitake mushroom, pomegranate, raspberry, reishi mushroom
Cankers	Goldenseal
Colds	Echinacea, andrographis, ginseng, coffee, licorice root (sore throat), tea (nasal and chest congestion)
Congestive heart failure	Hawthorn
Constipation	Apple, psyllium seed, senna
Cough	Eucalyptus
Depression	St. John's wort
Diabetes, Type 2	Garlic, beans (navy, pinto, black, etc.), cinnamon, eleutherococcus, flaxseed, green tea
Diabetic ulcers	Comfrey
Diarrhea	Bilberry, raspberry
Diverticulitis	Peppermint
Dizziness	Ginger, ginkgo
Earache	Echinacea
Eczema	Chamomile, topical borage seed oil, evening primrose oil
Fatigue	Cocoa (dark chocolate), coffee, eleutherococcus, ginseng, rhodiola, tea

Flu	Echinacea, elderberry syrup (also see "Colds")
Gas	Fennel, dill
Giardia	Goldenseal
Gingivitis	Goldenseal, green tea
Hay fever	Stinging nettle, butterbur
Herpes	Topical lemon balm, topical comfrey, echinacea, garlic, ginseng
High blood pressure	Garlic, beans, cocoa (dark chocolate), hawthorn
High blood sugar	Fenugreek
High cholesterol	Apple, cinnamon, cocoa (dark chocolate), evening primrose oil, flaxseed, soy foods, green tea
Hot flashes	Red clover, soy, black cohosh
Impotence	Yohimbe
Indigestion	Chamomile, ginger, peppermint
Infection	Topical tea tree oil, astragalus, echinacea, eleutherococcus, garlic, ginseng, rhodiola
Insomnia	Kava, evening primrose, hops, lemon balm, valerian
Irregular heartbeat	Hawthorn
Irregularity	Senna, psyllium seed
Irritable bowel syndrome	Chamomile, peppermint
Lower back pain	Thymol, carvacrol, white willow bark
Menstrual cramps	Kava, raspberry, chasteberry
Migraine	Feverfew, butterbur

Morning sickness	Ginger
Muscle pain	Capsicum, wintergreen
Nausea	Ginger
Premenstrual syndrome	Chasteberry, evening primrose
Ringing in the ears	Ginkgo
Seasonal affective disorder	St. John's wort
Shingles	Capsicum
Sore throat	Licorice, marshmallow, mullein
Stuffy nose	Echinacea
Tonsillitis	Goldenseal, astragalus, echinacea
Toothache	Willow, clove oil
Ulcers	Aloe, licorice
Varicosities	Bilberry, horse chestnut
Yeast infection	Garlic, goldenseal, pau d'arco

SOURCES

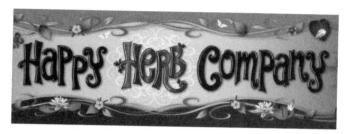

happyherbcompany.com

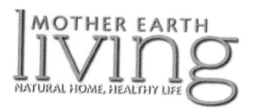

motherearthliving.com

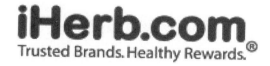

iherb.com

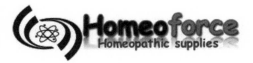

homeoforce.co.uk

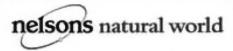

nelsonsnaturalworld.com

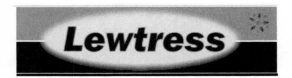

lewtress-health.com

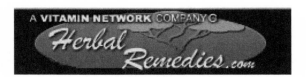

herbalremedies.com

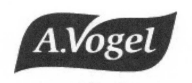

avogel.com

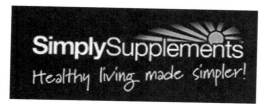

simplysupplements.net

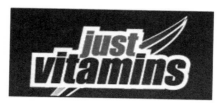

justvitamins.co.uk

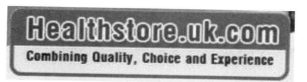

healthstore.uk.com

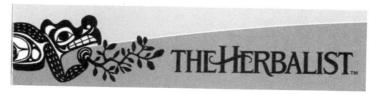

theherbalist.com

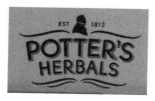

pottersherbals.co.uk

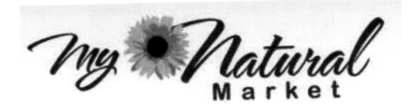

mynaturalmarket.com

HOLLAND & BARRETT

hollandandbarrett.com

FAQS

1. Is it okay to take herbal supplements along with antibiotics?

Although you must only take antibiotics when you really need them, there are times when only prescription medication will work. In this instance, you may wish to continue to take herbal remedies to assist your immune system in fighting off the bacteria. Probiotic supplements are great for reintroducing good bacteria, but you must consult your doctor first.

2. Are there any plants in the U.S. with antibiotic qualities that can be used externally?

There are many plants that grow in the U.S. with antibiotic qualities, and a selection of these can be used externally.

3. Are there any herbal remedies for (almost) chronic chest infections?

Official advice from NHS (nhs.uk/Conditions/Chest-infection-adult/Pages/Introduction.aspx) suggests that you can *help your body fight off the infection* by:

- Getting plenty of rest.

- Drinking lots of fluids to prevent dehydration and to thin the mucus in your lungs, making it easier to cough up.

- Treating headaches, fever, and aches and pains with painkillers such as paracetamol or ibuprofen.

- Drinking a warm drink of honey and lemon to relieve a sore throat caused by persistent coughing.

- Raising your head up with extra pillows while you sleep to make breathing easier.

- Using an air humidifier or inhaling steam from a bowl of hot water to ease your cough (hot water should not be used to treat young children with a cough due to the risk of scalds).

- Stopping smoking (if you smoke).

There are many online resources for finding suitable home remedies for anything, including chronic chest infections. Below is an *example for treating bronchitis*:

1. Mix half a teaspoon of ginger with half teaspoon each of pepper and cloves. This combination can be blended with a little honey to make it more palatable or consumed as a tea infusion. There are compounds in ginger, pepper, and cloves that help reduce fever and improve the immunity of the person suffering from bronchitis.

2. Add half a teaspoon of turmeric to a glass of milk and drink this three times a day. This natural remedy for bronchitis in children is more effective when taken on an empty stomach.

3. Infuse spinach leaves in water and add a pinch of honey and ammonium chloride. Drink this as a natural expectorant to loosen phlegm and reduce chest pain.

4. Powder the kernels of almonds and mix this powder in a glass of orange juice. Drink this every night before sleeping.

5. Use the powder of dry chicory root mixed in honey. You can get chicory root powder in most herbal or alternative medical stores. When taken three times daily, this is one of the most effective chronic bronchitis home remedies.

6. If you do suffer from shortness of breath or tightness in the chest, rubbing turpentine over the chest can offer some much-needed relief.

7. Warm salt water gargles can also help to loosen the phlegm and reduce constriction that you may feel in your chest.

8. The best way to treat bronchitis is by getting adequate rest. Doctors may prescribe an over-the-counter cough syrup to reduce the mucus buildup in your lungs. Cough drops can also reduce a sore throat but won't really stop the cough. In cases of chronic bronchitis or if you already suffer from a heart or lung disease, more medical attention and treatment will be necessary. Speak to your doctor immediately to prevent further medical complications.

4. What's the best natural antibiotic alternative to treat paronychia?

Paronychia is a common skin infection just next to the nail. Antibiotics are often prescribed for this, but there are natural alternatives available. Colloidal silver, Neosporin, and Sonoran are often recommended.

5. What is the most effective plant-based herbal antibiotic?

The most effective herbs are as follows:

- Grapefruit Seed Extract
- Echinacea
- Goldenseal
- Garlic
- Cranberry
- Uva Ursi
- Honey

All these herbs have been examined in detail in the 'Top 45 Wondrous Herbs' chapter.

6. How are antibiotics made and is it possible for a person to make their own?

Antibiotics are made by the process of fermentation. This is described in detail in the 'Usage of Antibiotics' chapter. It is possible for people to make their own antibiotics at home, and a few suitable recipes can be found in the 'Herbal Remedy Recipes' chapter.

7. Can I get rid of strep throat using herbal remedies instead of antibiotics?

Strep throat is a bacterial throat infection that makes your throat feel sore and scratchy. Herbal remedies are actually more beneficial for curing strep throat than antibiotics because the solution is more permanent. It is suggested that garlic, honey, and cayenne pepper are the best herbs for this issue.

8. Are there any herbal remedies for acne?

There are many herbal remedies that are useful for acne. It is suggested mixing the following ingredients, some of which need to be mixed with water, to form a face mask:

- Baking Soda
- Apple Cider Vinegar
- Coconut Oil
- Tea Tree Oil
- Egg Whites
- Lemon Juice

- Garlic (rub the slices on your skin)
- Ice Cubes
- Cornstarch
- Aloe

9. What is the best herbal treatment for cough?

There are lots of herbal remedies for coughs, but these are considered as *The Top 6:*

- A mix of honey, coconut oil, and lemon juice
- Thyme tea
- Black pepper and honey tea
- Lemon
- Licorice
- Ginger

10. What's the best herbal medicine for liver problems?

Herbal medicine has been used to help with liver problems for many years. Our modern day lifestyles put a lot of pressure on our liver, which is a problem because our liver is used for many vital functions – digestion, produces plasma proteins, stores iron, regulates the clotting of blood, synthesizes cholesterol, stores glucose as glycogen, regulates the levels of amino acids in blood, is involved with clotting of blood, removes toxins from the body, and produces immune factors that help prevent infections.

To keep our liver healthy, ***herbal remedies can be extremely beneficial.*** The following are suggested:

- Amla/Gooseberry – these are a great source of Vitamin C, and are used to help a sluggish liver.
- Jethimad/Licorice – these herbs are great for people who suffer from non-alcoholic fatty liver disease.
- Amrith/Guduchi – these are considered to have rejuvenating properties and help clear toxins out of the liver.
- Haldi/Turmeric – filled with valuable antioxidants and helps protect your liver.
- Flaxseeds – these help ease the strain on your liver.
- Vegetables – beets, cabbage, carrots, broccoli, onions, and garlic are great for helping the liver secrete greater concentrations of enzymes.

11. What is a good herbal remedy for allergies?

There are many brilliant herbal remedies that are suitable for allergies. The following are considered as *the most effective*:

- Butterbur – blocks the chemicals that block nasal passages.
- Quercetin – works as a cell stabilizer.
- Stinging Nettle – helps at the first sign of an allergic reaction.
- Bromelain – reduces nasal swelling and thins mucus.
- Phleum Pratense – reduces pollen allergy symptoms.
- Tinospora Cordifolia – reduces sneezing, itchiness, and nasal discharge.

12. Is there a way to cure eczema or dermatitis with herbal remedies?

Skin conditions such as eczema or dermatitis are cured easily with herbal remedies. In fact, there are so many available:

- Lactic acid bacteria as probiotics reduce the risk for infantile eczema.
- Evening primrose oil has therapeutic value in the treatment of atopic eczema.
- Exclusive breastfeeding reduces the incidence of atopic dermatitis in childhood.
- Topical Vitamin B-12 may be a treatment option in children with eczema.
- Fish oil supplementation in pregnancy and lactation may decrease the risk of infant allergy.
- Omega-3 fatty acids in breast milk protect against atopic eczema and allergic sensitization in infancy.
- TGF-beta in colostrum may prevent the development of atopic disease during exclusive breastfeeding and promote specific IgA production in human subjects.
- Vitamin D deficiency is higher among children with asthma, allergic rhinitis, atopic dermatitis, acute urticaria, and food allergy.
- Drinking deep-sea water restores mineral imbalance in atopic eczema/dermatitis syndrome.
- Oat and rice colloidal grain suspensions may safely be used as an adjunct in the management of mild atopic dermatitis in children under two years of age.

- Colloidal oatmeal may have value in the treatment of atopic dermatitis and other inflammatory and histamine-related conditions and may allow for reduced use of corticosteroids and calcineurin inhibitors.
- Black currant seed oil is well tolerated and transiently reduces the prevalence of atopic dermatitis in newborns.
- Borage oil is effective in treating atopic dermatitis.
- Topical St. John's wort cream may improve atopic dermatitis.
- Vitamin E and D supplementation improves symptoms of atopic dermatitis.
- A fermented whey protein and lactic acid bacteria complex has anti-inflammatory potential in an atopic dermatitis model.
- A traditional Korean fermented soybean food exhibits anti-inflammatory activity, which may have therapeutic value in allergic conditions such as asthma and atopic dermatitis.
- Kimchi contains a probiotic, Lactobacillus sakei, which alleviates allergen-induced skin inflammation in mice.
- Supplementation of Lactobacillus sakei in children with eczema-dermatitis syndrome is associated with a substantial clinical improvement.
- Probiotic supplementation may stabilize the intestinal barrier function and decrease gastrointestinal symptoms in children with atopic dermatitis.
- Supplementation of mothers and their babies with the probiotic Lactobacillus reuteri reduces IgE-associated eczema and may reduce respiratory allergic disease later in life.
- Supplementation with L. reuteri during late pregnancy reduces breast milk levels of TGF-beta2, which may be associated with less sensitization and possibly less IgE-associated eczema in breast-fed infants.
- Lactobacillus rhamnosus GG significantly reduces eczema in the first two years of life.
- Lactobacillus rhamnosus supplementation given to pregnant mothers and their offspring during the first six months of life is effective in preventing atopic disease in children at high risk.
- Probiotic and prebiotic supplementation improves the symptoms of children with atopic dermatitis.

- Bathing in a magnesium-rich Dead Sea salt solution improves skin barrier function, enhances skin hydration, and reduces inflammation in atopic dry skin.

- White rose petal extract has anti-allergic and anti-atopic properties.

13. Which herbal antibiotics can be taken during pregnancy?

You always need to check with your doctor before taking herbal supplements when pregnant. Due to the lack of regulation, it is always advisable to get the opinion of a medical professional. These are considered as the *safest herbal antibiotics*:

- Garlic
- Coconut Oil
- Grapefruit Seed Extract
- Cranberry
- Colloidal Silver
- Shatavari
- Vitamins D, C, and A

14. How do herbal antibiotics fight bacteria?

Natural antibiotics operate in two primary ways. First of all, they eliminate the dangerous germs. One of the disadvantages is that they can kill some helpful bacteria as well, but that is considered a tiny price to pay if you compare the final results of the proliferation of those germs within your body. Nevertheless, the quantity of helpful microorganisms that is wiped out tends to be exceptionally small. Additionally, their performance is far superior if you compare them with the quantity of useful bacteria killed by artificial antibiotics.

The second way in which these natural alternatives to antibiotics work is by boosting the body's defenses. In this way, your body system will be capable of fighting back any germs and their consequences. The advantage with this strategy is that no helpful bacteria will be eradicated.

Essentially, natural antibiotics are a great way to boost your overall health and eliminate harmful bacteria from your body.

CONCLUSION

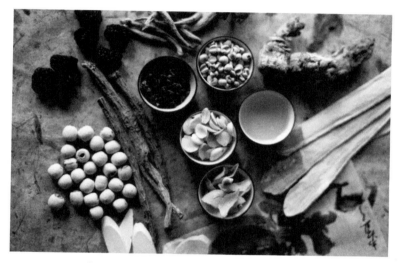

So as you can see from this book, herbal antibiotics are a great alternative to conventional medicine when it comes to helping your body fight off bacterial infections. They have fewer side effects; they have a much more widespread availability and, ensuring that you only use traditional antibiotics when you need them, reduce the risk of antibiotic resistance.

There are many ways that you can consume these natural antibiotics. Of course, there are the tablets, medicines, and oils, but there are also a lot of food, herbs, and spices that can be incorporated into your everyday diet to ensure you are always protected. After all, there can't be any downsides to making your body healthier and better able to fight anything that threatens it! Of course, you will need to consult your doctor to confirm that any of the herbal and natural remedies are suitable for you, but once you have made the lifestyle change, you won't want to go back.

ABOUT THE AUTHOR

Mary Jones became interested in herbal remedies early on in her life. After becoming frustrated with the ineffectiveness and sometimes severe side effects of synthetic remedies, she started researching whether or not natural cures could be made to the same effect, without the use of synthetic means. After dedicating years of her life to research, learning from natural remedies masters, as well as from doctors that use natural cures to help their patients, she decided it was time to share the knowledge she had gathered with the world.

One of Mary's life goals is to make the world a better, happier place, and her writings are definitely a testament to that. She has not just kept all of her research and discoveries to herself. She has elected to share them, in a format that makes them available to just about everyone. And instead of talking about just the unknown or difficult-to-find herbs as many naturalists do, she has selected remedies that anyone can make, so that every person can make themselves healthier, easily and inexpensively. Mary's books aren't just about theory; they are about practice – actually fighting infections and ailments naturally!